I0752257

A Simplified and Sometimes Sassy Guide to Breast Cancer

For more resources: sassybreastcancerguide.com

Library of Congress Control Number

ISBN paperback: 978-1-7373793-3-1

eBook ISBN: 978-1-7373793-0-0

Cover Design and Book Design by: Brittany Mathias, MD

Graphics and Illustrations: Vectors provided by graphicmama.com and edited by Brittany Mathias, MD unless otherwise noted.

Printed in the United States of America

A Simplified and Sometimes Sassy Guide to Breast Cancer

Like if your best friend was a breast surgeon

Brittany Mathias, MD

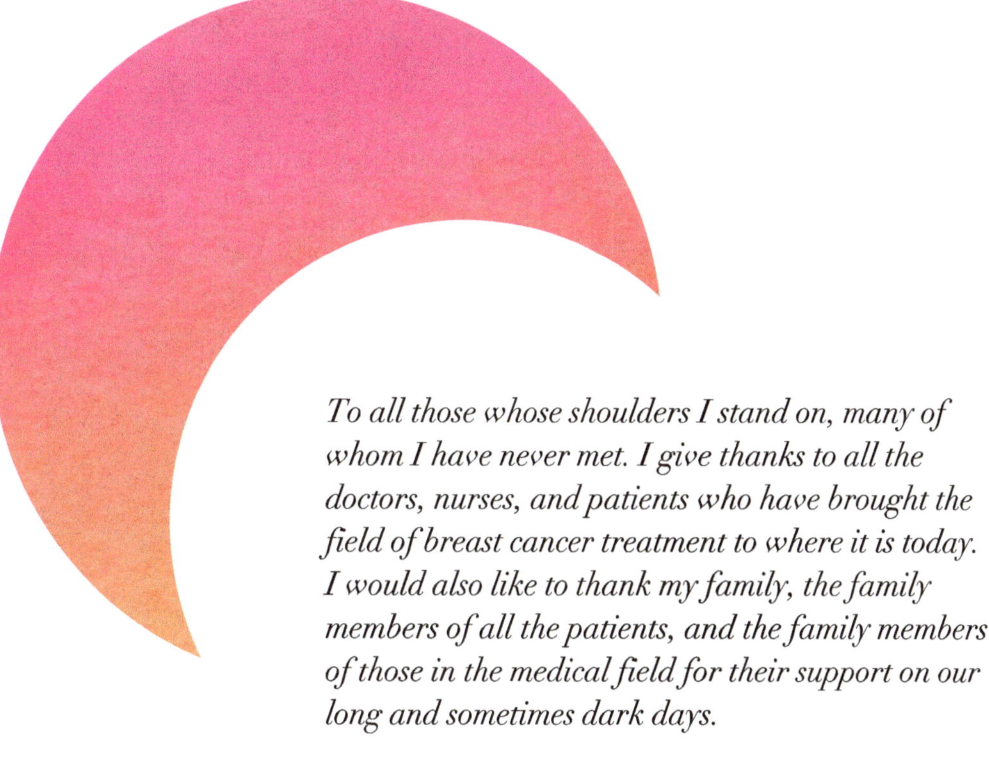

To all those whose shoulders I stand on, many of whom I have never met. I give thanks to all the doctors, nurses, and patients who have brought the field of breast cancer treatment to where it is today. I would also like to thank my family, the family members of all the patients, and the family members of those in the medical field for their support on our long and sometimes dark days.

I wanted to write this book as a gift of both understanding and companionship. My goal is to arm you with the knowledge you need to cast aside the anxiety that comes from the unknown and help you make the right decision for YOU! You do not have to go through this alone. My greatest hope is that this book will be a little ray of sunshine on an otherwise cloudy day. I want you to have the best chance to succeed so that you can place this whole mess behind you and get on with LIFE!

Brittany Mathias, MD

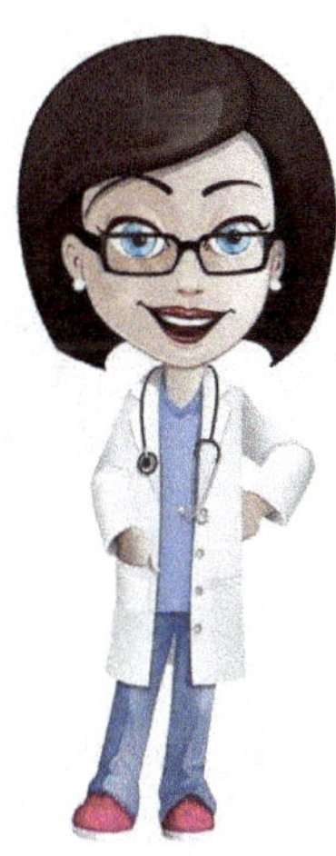

Table of

Contents

Forward Dr. Alan Hollingsworth

1 *Introduction* 3

Illustration Guide
Is This my Fault? Heck No!
What is Cancer Anyway? Well...

2 *The A-Team* 12

The Who's Who of Your Fab Team

3 *Radiology* 18

I've Never Taken So Many Pictures of My Boobs!

4 *Pathology* 32

Ouch! Someone Poked Me!

5 *Surgery* 46

I Am I Going to Lose My Breasts?
"Oncoplastic Reconstruction after Lumpectomy" by Dr. Maryann Martinovic

6 *Radiation* 92

A Day at the Beach
"Brachytherapy, What Is It?" by Astrid Morrison, M.D.
"Heart Disease and Radiation" by Dr. David Schomas

7 *Medical Oncology* *114*

Bartender!

8 *Special Cases* 140

I'm Pregnant - Help!
Inflammatory Breast Cancer - My Breast Is Red!
Paget's Disease - My Nipple Looks Weird!
Phyllodes

9 *Stage IV* 144

My Cancer Flew the Coop!

10 *Timeline* 148

Break it Down!

11 *Alternative Therapy* 152

Crystals, Herbs, and Some Gal in Mexico

12 *Genetics* 156

Who Am I Really?

13 *Survivorship* 160

I Jumped Through Fire, Tamed Lions . . .
"What To Do Next?" by DeBorrah Carter

14 *Clinical Trials* 170

Do I Need One?

15 *Do I Need a Second Opinion?* 174

Or a Third?

16 *Resources* 176

I Need More!

17 *Good Luck Girlfriend!* *178*

You Can Do It!

18 *Expert Extras* 179

In Case You Needed a Little More . . .

"A Detailed and Debated Debrief on MRI"
by Dr. Alan Hollingsworth

"Lymphedema"
by Dr. Lisa Spiguel

"Bras and Prosthetics and Posture, Oh My!"
by Victoria Hand

"Proton Therapy"
by Dr. Schomas

19 *Glossary* 193

Foreword

Over 300,000 times every year in the US alone, these words are strung together in one fashion or another: "Your biopsy results show that you have breast cancer." And with that, lives are changed forever.

In the past, this change meant disfiguring surgery at an absolute minimum, giving a unique aspect to breast cancer when compared to other types of malignancy—visibility. That is, the patient (and any significant other) could see the havoc wreaked from treatment, unlike most other types of cancer where surgical tracks can be neatly tucked away inside the body. Breast cancer was, therefore, a one-two punch; it brought mutilation and the possibility of death.

By the 1980s, however, things began to change. Breast conservation (lumpectomy) with radiation emerged as an alternative to mastectomy, while at the same time, the introduction of screening mammography facilitated this change by identifying smaller tumors. The idea of administering "adjuvant" chemotherapy or endocrine therapy after tumor removal, without proven metastatic disease, was a new concept, readily adopted when it became clear that more lives were being saved. The vast majority of women today will beat breast cancer, largely through earlier diagnosis as well as these "adjuvant" systemic therapies. The introduction of endocrine therapy using tamoxifen was a major development at this same time, sparing many women aggressive surgical procedures used through the 1970s, such as removal of the adrenal glands or the pituitary, designed to lower hormone levels as much as possible. And with the introduction of breast implants to reconstruct patients after mastectomy, another specialist entered the breast cancer treatment group—the plastic surgeon.

What was missing, however, was communication among the multiple specialists who were crossing each other's pathways and burning each other's bridges. Today, we take the multidisciplinary approach to breast cancer for granted. But there was a time when specialists did not communicate well. Even after the introduction of breast conservation, it was commonly heard: "I tell the patient why she should have a mastectomy, then I send her to the radiation oncologist who tells her why she should have a lumpectomy. Then, she decides."

Gradually, the multidisciplinary conference emerged, not only involving all the treating specialists, but also the radiologist who read the breast imaging studies and the pathologist who interpreted the slides because, as it turned out, the diagnostic challenges could be as difficult as the treatment plan. Nonetheless, clinicians learned to sit at the same table and communicate.

In addition to facilitating patient care, something else happened when everyone gathered in the same room—the specialists educated each other. Prone to read only the medical journals pertaining to one's specialty, surgeons in the conference setting learned about radiation oncology studies, medical oncologists listened to advances in surgical approaches, and so forth. Today, in those hospitals with high-volume breast cancer management, colleagues are so attuned to the other specialists on the team that they can nearly recite each other's literature and treatment plans.

But something else happened as we entered the new millennium—extreme complexity regarding options. It was no longer a matter of mastectomy vs. lumpectomy. There were different ways to approach mastectomy, different ways to reconstruct, different approaches to lymph node evaluation (sentinel node biopsy), different ways to perform conservation ("oncoplastics"), different methods of radiation, different options to the "old standard" tamoxifen, different chemotherapeutic agents, different order of treatment modalities (neoadjuvant therapy), not to mention different classification schemes devised for breast cancer pathology, a different staging system, different imaging modalities to help with pre-operative planning . . . You get the picture!

In all the muddle, the patient can get lost. So, in this book written by breast-dedicated surgeon, Brittany Mathias, MD, we have a candid look at the complexity of options, clarified nicely in a frank, sometimes humorous approach (yes, there is humor after breast cancer) that pulls the reader in like a good novel. In the pages of this "Introduction to Breast Cancer Options 101" style book, the newly diagnosed breast cancer patient is presented with a wonderful overview to help in the decision-making process.

As a breast-dedicated surgeon for many years, I always intended to write a book like this, but it never made it off my to-do list. Just as well, because Dr. Mathias has filled the void with this entertaining look at the many issues and controversies facing the newly diagnosed breast cancer patient. And she did it with sister-to-sister charm and more wit than I could have managed. This is a must-read book for the newly diagnosed breast cancer patient.

Alan B. Hollingsworth, MD

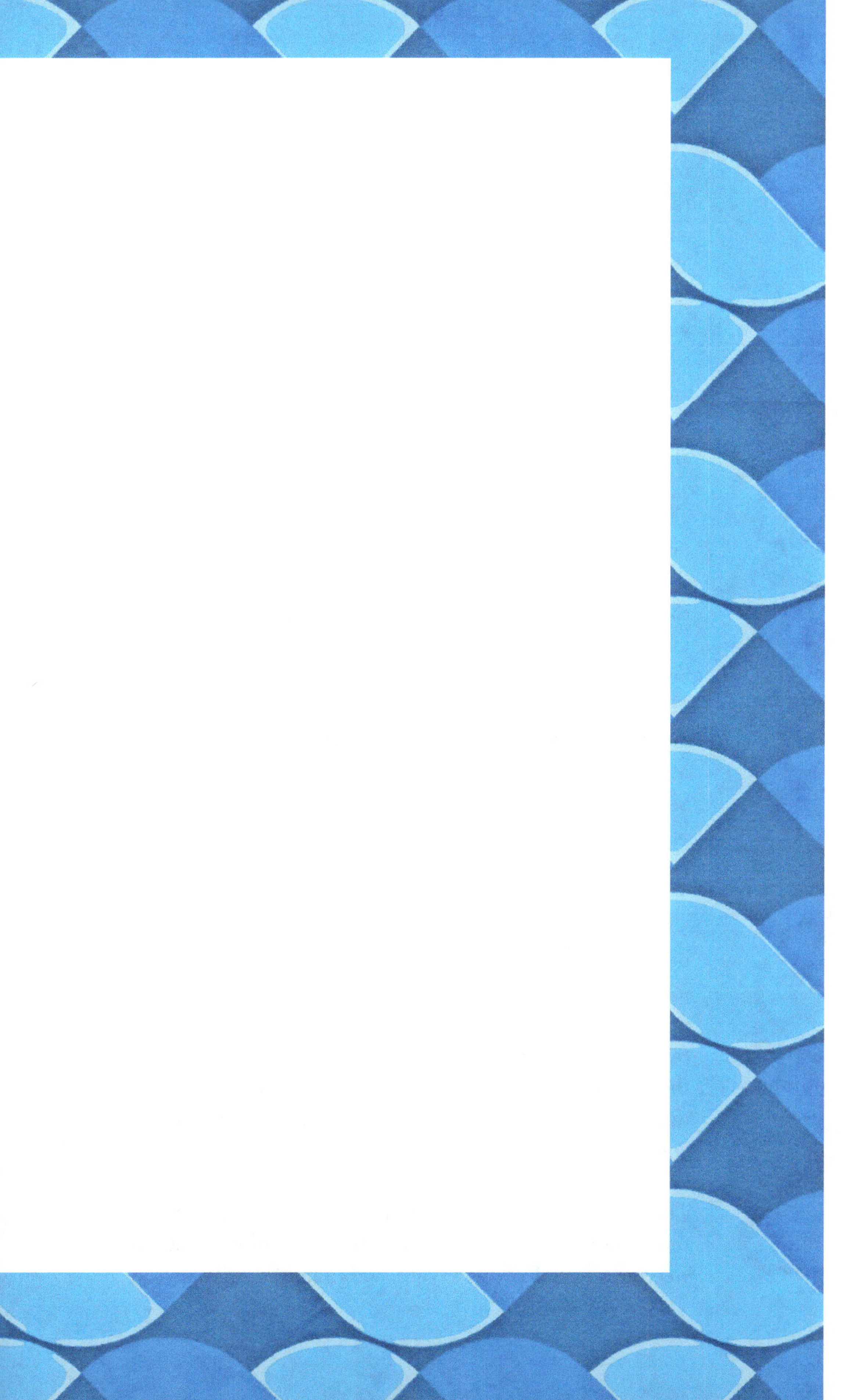

Welcome!

We aren't sugarcoating this one and telling ourselves half-truths. Nope, not this time, princess. We are going into this with knowledge. We are going to keep our heads high and our hopes high because the odds are on your side! You are reading this because the unknown is scary stuff. If we can just put it all on the table, we will know what we are dealing with and then begin to tackle one thing at a time! Remember, you have just joined a sisterhood of amazing and resilient strong women. One in eight women will get breast cancer in their lifetime, so you are not alone.

This book is no substitute for the rockstar team of doctors, nurses, and support staff who will help you along the way. But it is a great way to lay the groundwork for the many conversations to come. It will also work to fill in the details that your curious mind will ask at 3:00 a.m. but will absolutely not remember when the doctor says, "Do you have any questions?" Frankly, it's not easy to digest the massive amount of information you will get over the next several days, weeks, and months. There will be a ton of new information and a ton of treatment options, and all of this will be given to you in a whole new language (the cancer lingo).

So, let's do this! You may want to read each chapter before each specialist's office visit. You may want to read it in one night and highlight it—jot questions in the margins and earmark pages. You may feel completely overwhelmed, throw this book at a wall, and let it sit there for a few days because—damn it—"I can't deal with this!" You do you! We all learn differently, and we all cope differently.

This might even be the time to get into your car, turn up the music, drive down the street, and yell while hitting the steering wheel. I'm just saying . . . No judgment here.

Illustration Guide

Throughout this book, there are illustrations to help all the visual learners out there! Let's meet our merry band of characters!

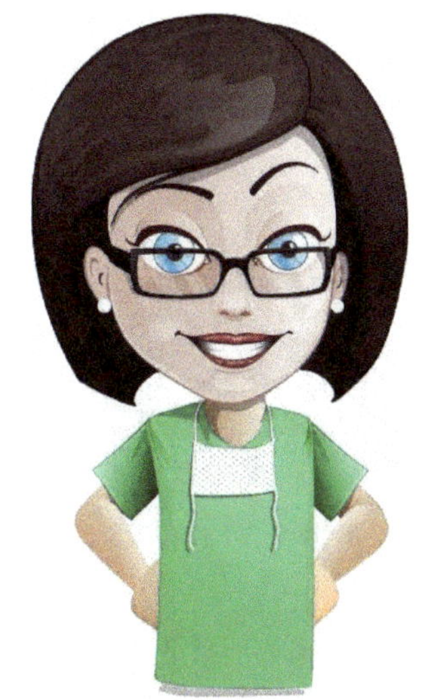

Our Gal!
She is our stand-in for doc, friend, & patient.

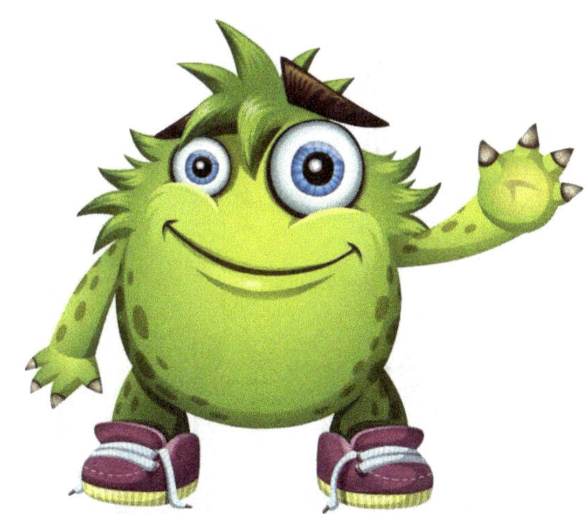

Cancer Cell

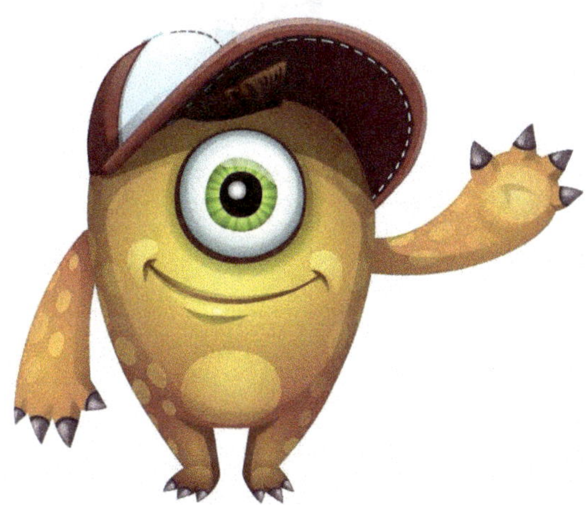

Lymph Node

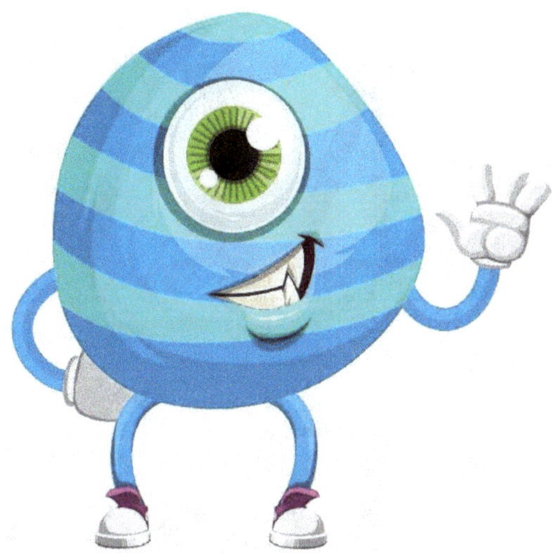

Healthy Body Cell

There are also special sections within each chapter: science bits, history bits, and expert bits. If it doesn't interest you, skip these and circle back later, if desired. I have placed the bulk of the expert bits in the back because these fantastic people get into some serious detail. I hope you can unpack these deeper dives once you've completed this book and determined which topics best pertain to you.

Is This My Fault?

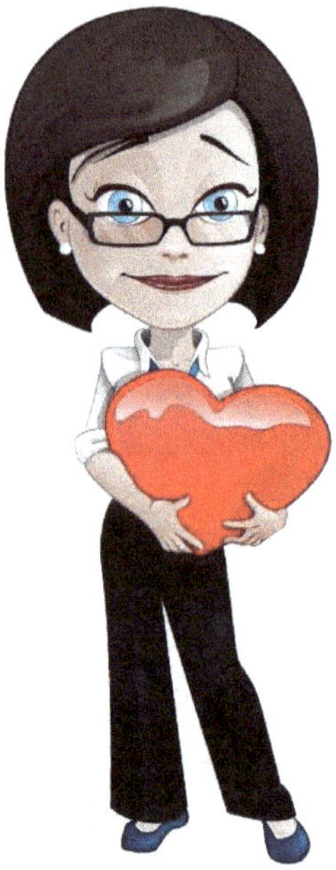

Heck No!

If you are trying to place blame reading about risk factors online . . . knock it off! The biggest risk factor is being female, and you didn't do anything to deserve this. If you are trying to blame that glass of wine, a few extra pounds, not getting pregnant at a younger age, not breastfeeding long enough (or at all), or taking hormone replacement pills that rescued you from the pits of menopause hell, then I'm here to say, "Sister! Pump those blame breaks!" I have seen women who don't smoke or drink with a BMI (body mass index) of sixteen who are vegan and run marathons with AA cup-sized breasts get cancer. Remember, breast cancer occurs in one in eight women!

Risk factors are population based. There is no way to go back in time and change things now. And frankly, even if you did, there's no proving that it would change anything. Take that pointing finger, give your hand a good shake, shut your eyes, and have a "Good Will Hunting" moment. That means give yourself a hug and repeat after me: "It's not my fault." (Good Will Hunting is a 1997 movie starring Matt Damon. If you haven't seen it, it's worth watching!) Anyway, what is important is that we have found this doggone cancer, and now we can assemble a team of helpers and take action! Hurrah!

What Is Cancer Anyway?

Well . . .

Cancer is simple and it's complex. The way I like to think about it will, of course, involve food! Recall that great cookie recipe in your grandma's handwriting. Everything is going great until you are squinting and wondering, Is that tablespoons or teaspoons? And let's face it, she made her cookies from memory without measuring cups, so there's no way that your cookies are going to turn out the same as her cookies. Then, maybe your friend wants the recipe, and you transcribe it in your own creative cursive scrawl. And "oh boy!" we are on the path to getting into a heap of chocolate-chip trouble. Those perfect cookies are morphing into salty, flat blobs.

Well, our bodies do this every day when they make new cells. DNA is the recipe, literally copied one letter at a time, and the cookies are our cells. While our bodies have many safety checks to fix poorly copied recipes, mistakes happen!

Those bad cookies can become self-destructive little bombs that go kapow! and kill themselves (think of cookies burnt beyond all recognition), or they can alert the immune system (the baker tastes a batch and chucks those cookies in the trash), or they can grow and grow . . . and grow. Those are the troublemakers, the super sneaky, salty cookies that otherwise looked great, so you gift-wrapped and gave them to all your friends before you actually tasted one; those are the cancer cookies.

To summarize, cancer is like a bad cookie resulting from a bad recipe. It's the recipe that determines how nasty these cookies are. This is similar to hearing your doctor talk about "favorable biology" (nice cancer) or "bad biology" (aggressive cancer). We have some ways to determine just how bad these cookies are. Think receptors, Oncotype Dx score®, evidence of travel, and so on. If all that jargon piqued your anxiety, don't worry! I will eventually demystify this terminology. But first, there is still a lot we don't know that only time, and a lot of science, will tell. Don't turn to doctor Google to decode that last sentence. Instead, take a deep breath and move on! Remember, each of these things will be discussed in more detail as we get to them!

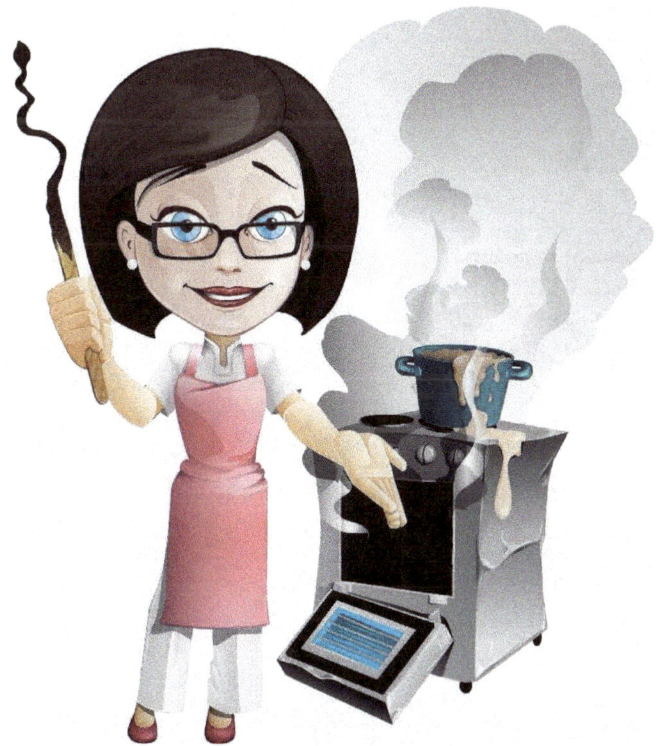

Yeast

Okay, so you are trying to grasp the cookies/cancer schtick. But you decide, "Nah, it's not for me." A slightly more accurate comparison would be a sourdough yeast starter.

Has a friend ever baked you some magical, fantastic bread and then offered you a "starter." These are usually gifted in a plastic bag or a mason jar with a list of instructions on feeding and dividing your starter and baking your bread. This can be some labor-intensive stuff!

If you don't appropriately maintain and divide this concoction or get an accurate recipe, then you're not going to end up with warm, yummy bread. It's the same idea with cancer in the body; you need good directions (DNA) and a good starter (a healthy cell).

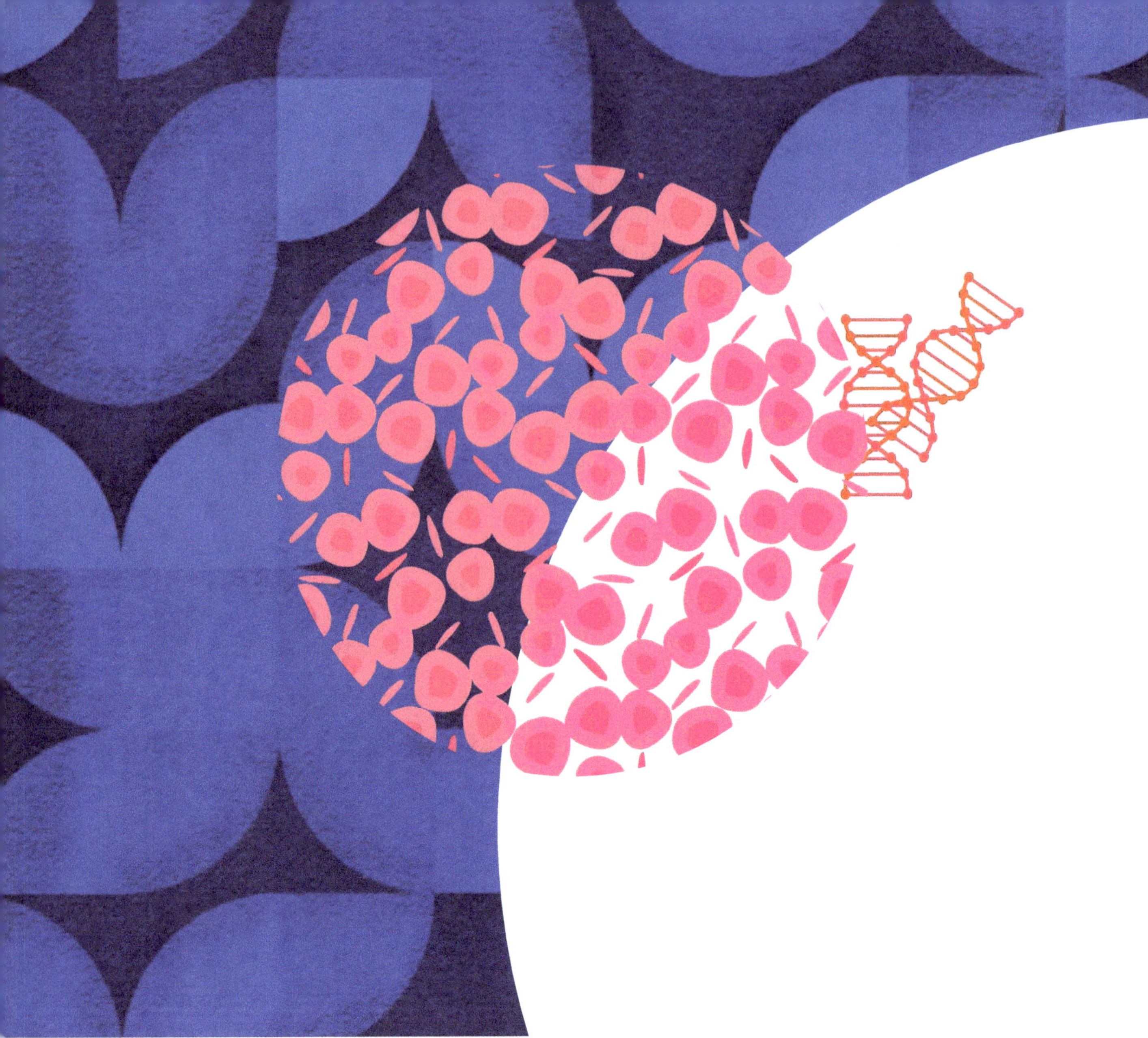

SCIENCE SIMPLIFIED!

Throughout this book, there will be "science simplified" sections. For those of you who are totally and completely overwhelmed right now, feel free to skip these! The science sections are for you curious cats that just need to know more. You are the ladies that are always asking, "How does that work?" and "Why do I have to do that?" These little asides are for you. My goal is to answer those questions on the molecular level and to simplify some pretty hefty science so that you know what is going on!

First, a little more on DNA. Behold our human body recipe: the DNA double helix. DNA is written in a very simple code with only four letters (ACGT). These guys come in pairs; A and T are best buddies, and C and G are best buddies! From this simple recipe comes you! The goods and what I affectionately call the others (no negative self-talk here ladies!). If you unwound all this DNA and placed it end to end, you'd find that each individual cell contains about six feet of DNA. Instead of having six feet of continuous DNA, the body chops it into pieces (called chromosomes) and winds it up in places like little spools of thread. We have twenty-three chromosomes and two copies of each chromosome. One copy comes from dad, and one copy comes from mom, which gives you a total of forty-six chromosomes. That's a ton of information, but interestingly, the "genes" only make up about 3 percent of this information—3 percent! (Think about the genes as the ingredient list and all the other stuff as the instructions.) Some genes are huge (millions of ACG and Ts), and some are small (a few hundred ACG and Ts).

The BRCA1 gene, for instance, is 81,188 base pairs long (a base pair is one letter with its best buddy). If you are born with an error in this gene, you may have an increased risk of breast cancer and ovarian cancer.

We will dive deeper into genetics and risks later. We usually think of our DNA as the thing that sets us apart and makes us different. Incredibly, we all share about 99.9 percent of our DNA. Wowza!

Words from Your Sisters:

You are not alone!

I did a ton of research before I made a decision. The team had to be one could I work with and make decisions *with*.

Survivor Sister

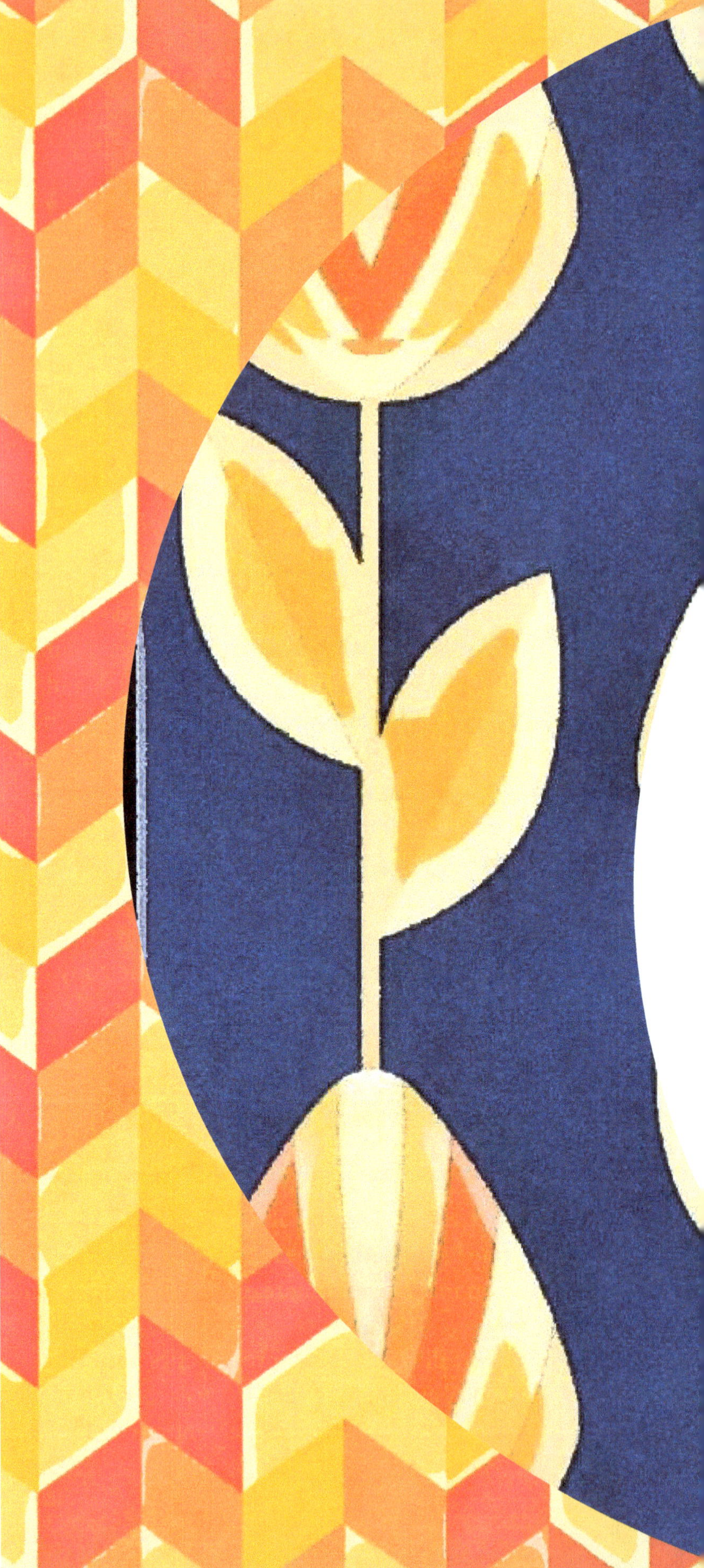

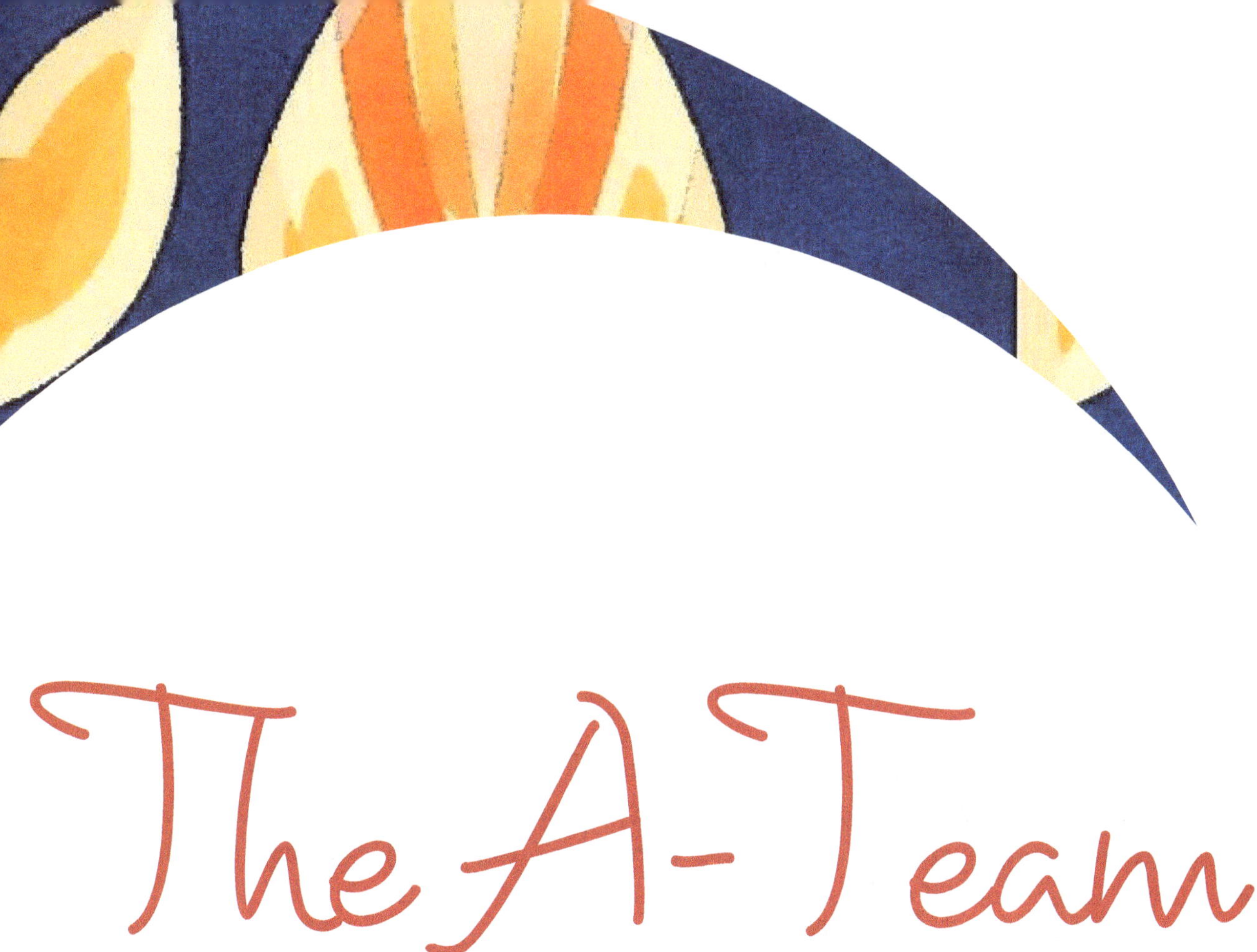

The A-Team

Here's the bottom line: your doctors have traveled an incredibly long road to have the privilege to take care of you! Thank you for letting us be a part of the answers to your questions, a shoulder for you to cry on, and, hopefully, the solution to what ails you! Here's a rundown on who these people are and how they got here.

Radiologist

This is likely the first doctor you will meet after the mammogram or at that really—ouch!—wonderful biopsy. They like dark rooms and physics, but we certainly won't hold that against them. For those of you who have experienced a mammogram, these fantastic people can interpret something that looks like a TV snowstorm when the signal's gone out. They're so sharp, they can find a cancer as small as three millimeters! They completed four years of college, four years of medical school, one year of internship, four years of radiology residency, and many spend an extra year in breast radiology fellowship.

Surgical Oncologist

Often this is the next doctor you meet after your radiologist. These guys and gals have completed four years in college, four years in medical school, five years in general surgery residency (taking out cancers all over the body, dealing with mass trauma, working thirty-six-hour shifts), and in some cases, a surgical oncology fellowship (two years for specialization in cancer all over the body) or a breast surgical oncology fellowship (one year doing all things related to breasts—breast medical oncology, breast radiation oncology, breast pathology, etc.). Along the way, many surgeons do one or more years of research in a lab with PhDs, taking a deeper dive into the science side of medicine.

Plastic Surgeon

While we are talking surgeons, a good number of you will also meet a plastic surgeon. Most breast surgeons partner with a plastic surgeon. The breast surgeon removes the cancer and takes into consideration the cancer aspect of the surgery. Then, the plastic surgeon comes in and crafts some new breasts or can even reduce and lift what you have left. (Yes, you could end up with perkier breasts at the end of this!) They have completed four years of college, four years of medical school, and either five years of general surgery residency followed by three years of plastic surgery fellowship or six years of plastic surgery residency. Then some will go on to complete fellowships one to two years in length. And, of course, they may have done some science research too!

Medical Oncologist

You will likely meet one of these wonderful people. They will hold your hand through the good and the bad for the long haul—decades sometimes. They are incredibly optimistic and supportive. They completed four years of college, four years of medical school, three years of medicine residency (taking care of just about any inpatient medical issue . . . think heart attacks, pneumonia, and, of course, cancer), then three or more years of hematology/oncology fellowship specializing in blood diseases and cancer-related illness. Some of them do an extra year of fellowship in breast medical oncology. And again, some of them take a deep dive into science research with a PhD for one or more years.

Radiation Oncologist

These professionals have an incredible capacity for physics and math despite also being part of patient care. They completed four years of college, four years of medical school, one year of internship, and four years of radiation oncology residency. They also do more than dabble in some pretty advanced physics; these lads and ladies spent numerous hours in the library during training as they require a dubious "record" four board certification examinations: Clinical Oncology, Radiation Biology, Radiation Physics, and a summary Oral Board.

Pathologist

You won't meet these unsung heroes. They look at cells under microscopes all day. Just like those fantastic radiologists reading the snowstorm, these team players interpret pink and purple abstract art all day. Now if you are thinking all "cell stuff" looks the same, then you'll understand why pathologists spend so many years honing their skills so they can give us the answers we need. They completed four years of college, four years of medical school, four years of pathology residency, followed—in some cases—by one year of breast pathology fellowship.

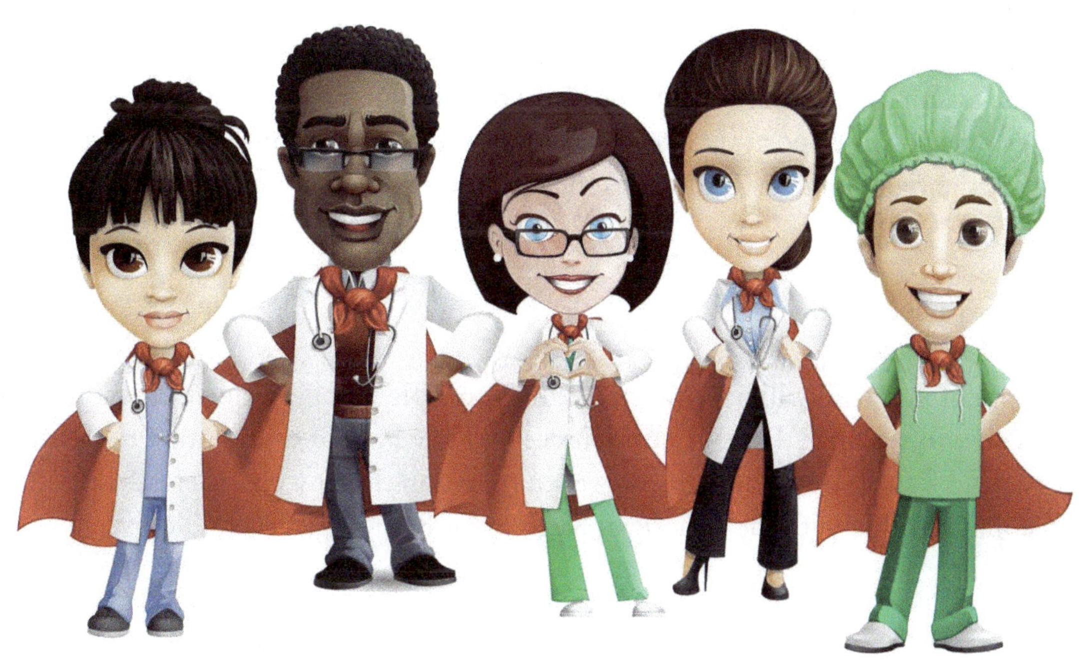

Nurse Navigator

Depending on where you get your care, you may be lucky enough to have one of these people on your team. They are the point person for it all! They help coordinate appointments with your doctors, cut through insurance red tape, lobby for financial assistance if you need it, and help you find your support group sisters! Most cancer centers have these "can-do" people. (Frankly, I don't know how I would function without one!)

Genetic Counselor

These highly specialized people have completed four years of college, followed by a master's degree in genetic counseling. They know their stuff! If you do end up having some genetic variants, they will counsel you on all "the things" that will be tailored for you and your family—from extra screening recommendations to preventative surgery options. Don't have one at your hospital? No problem, they can also be found on the other end of a video chat or phone call.

Physician Assistants and Advanced Registered Nurse Practitioners

These guys and gals arrive here by all sorts of roads. The bottom line is that they spent some good time getting extra education to help you (undergraduate degrees and post-graduate training)! You may encounter these people along the way as they lend an ear, provide emotional support, pull your drains, or see you at follow-up appointments. They are the right hand of the doctors they partner with, and they are great people.

Radiation Therapist

For those of you who will have radiation, these people will become your fast friends since you will see them daily for several weeks. They have keen attention to detail too! They spend four years obtaining a degree in radiation therapy and then take the steps to become certified with the American Registry of Radiologic Technologists.

Support Staff

They make it all possible! A special nod to the medical assistants, schedulers, front desk staff, hospital staff, nurses, cleaning staff, security guards, and so many others. Doctors are only able to help you because these people help us!

Patient Navigators and Support Groups

You are not alone! There is likely a support group in your area with women who have been in your shoes. If you feel that you need some community, then reach out! If there is not a group in your area, there are always online groups too. Just remember that everyone's journey is unique to them, and the right answer for someone else may not be the right answer for you.

At some of the larger cancer centers, you might also have access to a patient navigator. These ladies have had cancer and have taken some extra time learning about breast cancer in order to serve as peer support with some extra knowledge. You can ask your nurse navigator if your institution has any of these lovely ladies available to chat.

The Home Team

Don't forget to rally the home team! Now is the time to establish your Survivor Support Team! Who will drive you to and from the hospital? Who will run to the pharmacy? Who will call the doctor at 2:00 a.m. even when you really don't think it's necessary? Invite these people into your world! You certainly don't need to shout, "I have breast cancer!" from the rooftops or hold an HOA meeting. But, you are going to need some family or friends or neighbors . . . or maybe a little bit of everyone who loves you. Remember that you have people in your life who want to be there for you. It may be hard to let them in and ask for favors, but when you are ready, make them part of your team.

Words from Your Sisters:

You are not alone!

The information that you are given is like a thunderstorm coming at you. It's overwhelming. I have a medical background, and I truly have no idea how women can navigate the medical system when confronted with this diagnosis. This was one of the hardest parts of the journey, the decision-making part. You need to take a deep breath, get the information, and then make a decision on how to move forward with a treatment plan by talking with people you trust and love.

Survivor Sister

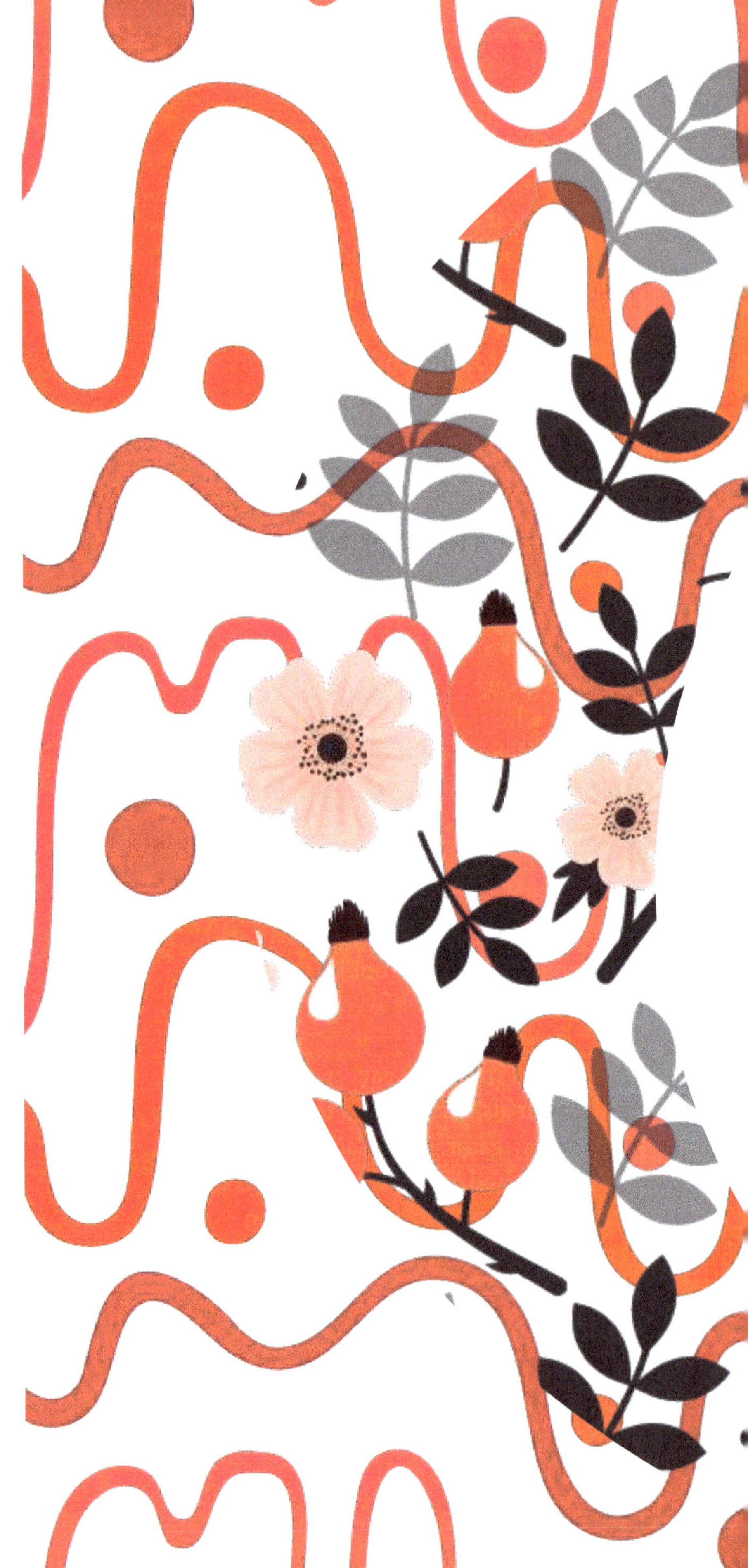

Radiology

I've Never Taken So Many Pictures of My Boobs!

Someone has just told you that there's a mass and—boom!—your mind goes blank, your thoughts swim haphazardly, and you cannot remember anything else that they said afterward. How could you be expected to keep a level head? Well, if you are holding your radiology report, take a deep breath. Maybe let out a long "om" if you're into that, or say a little prayer for strength. Once you're a bit more grounded, skip to the "IMPRESSION" section at the bottom of the radiology report for the synopsis. Here's where the paragraphs above will be summarized and interpreted. And the next thing you will see will be the BI-RADS score. Yes, you are learning a new language. BI-RADS stands for Breast Imaging-Reporting and Data System.

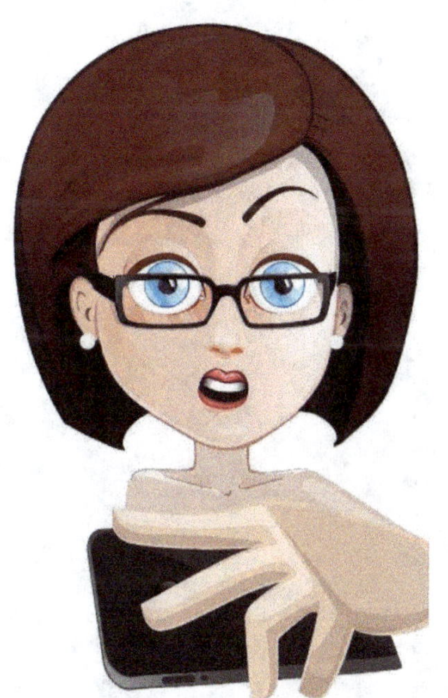

BI-RADS

The first thing to understand about your radiology reports is the BI-RADS system. This is a score that every breast image gets (it doesn't matter if it's a mammogram, breast MRI, or breast ultrasound) to classify the findings and help decide the next course of action. Now, you need to realize that the BI-RADS Atlas is hundreds of pages long (and it is extremely specific!). But here are the basics.

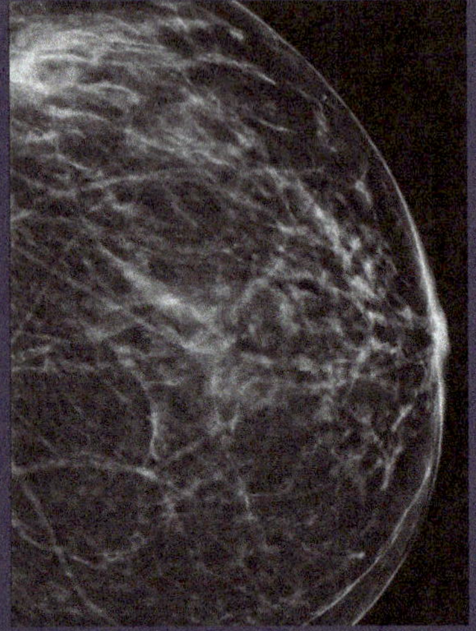

BI-RADS 1

You may have seen one of these in the past. Decoded, it means, "That is one normal, no bad-business breast. See you in one year. Tata for now, ta-tas!"

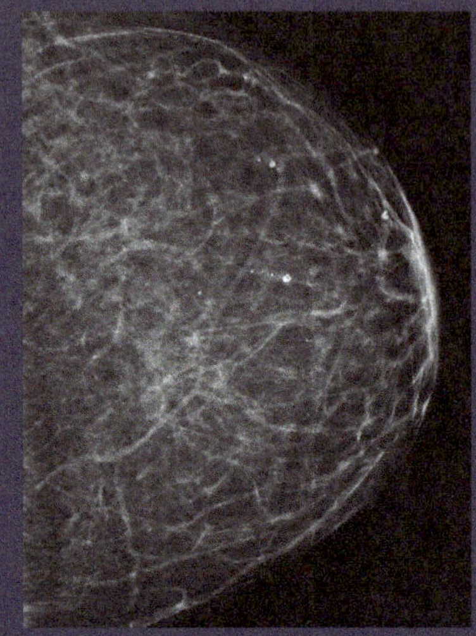

BI-RADS 2

There is certainly something there, but let's not worry about that little thang! This is the stuff that's been showing up consistently without change. It can represent a lot of different things—from benign breast business to scars from prior surgery. At the end of the day, it is the stuff that's clearly benign or normal. But since it's still there, we will acknowledge it.

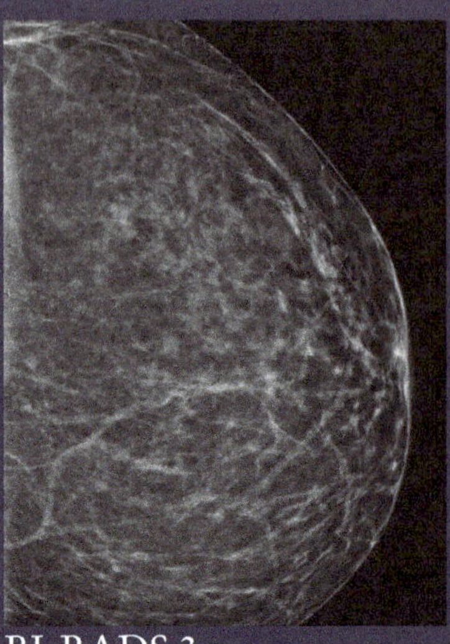

BI-RADS 3

Hmm. We are pretty sure that's not cancer (that means that there's a less than 2 percent chance it's cancer). There is no need to biopsy it now, but let's take another look at it in six months, please. Let's not wait a year. If you have some "other" spots on your breasts that are given a BI-RADS 3, you and your surgeon may decide to biopsy this thing now or factor that little spot into your surgical planning.

BI-RADS **0**

This means "incomplete." Anyone who found their cancer on a screening mammogram got one of these and was then called back for more imaging (that first "holey guacamole moment"). It means that "something" was found and additional images are needed to assign a true BI-RADS score. These will become BIRADS 2, 3, 4, and 5 with further imaging.

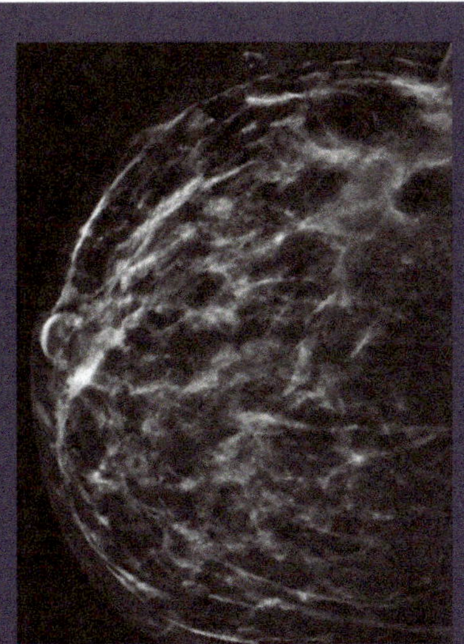

BI-RADS 4

Yowza! Let's biopsy that, pronto! We don't like the look of this image, and it could be cancer. BI-RADS 4 is sometimes broken down further into 4a, 4b, and 4c. 4a has a 13 percent chance of being cancer; 4b a 36 percent chance of being cancer; and 4c a 79 percent chance of being cancer. All comers to the group have about a 30 percent chance of finding cancer when a biopsy is performed. But let's be real: for you, it was all or nothing.

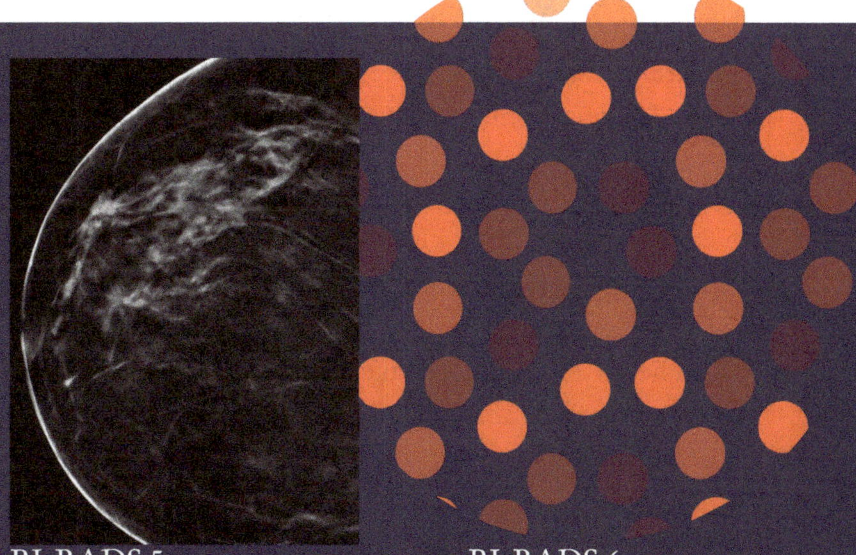

BI-RADS 5

Girl, that's cancer (about 95 percent of the time). And while we need some pathology (tissue from a biopsy) to prove it and help devise a plan, we are pretty darn sure of the diagnosis. Full steam ahead!

BI-RADS 6

Well, we know it's cancer. We have the pathology to prove it, but we need more imaging (think about that breast MRI you may have had or the additional ultrasounds performed after the MRI). These get a BI-RADS 6, so everyone reading the report knows that there is a known cancer.

Okay, now we have our

All Photos Courtesy of Melanie Pearce, DO

scoring system. There are three main ways we image breasts and the lymph nodes in the armpits. And I know you are certainly not a stranger to breast imaging at this point. If you think someone is taking you for a ride, trying to get multiple mammograms, ultrasounds, breast MRIs, and repeat ultrasounds, fear not; this is sometimes just a part of the process. Each type of imaging has its advantages and disadvantages. And realize, too, that every kind of imaging will come up with a different size for your cancer. That's to be expected. No, your cancer did not grow from 1.2 cm (on the ultrasound you had one week ago) to 2.0 cm (on the MRI you had today).

Mammogram: It's an X-ray of the Breast

This heavy hitter is a lifesaver! Screening mammograms have decreased death from breast cancer by about 40 percent! Let's give a round of applause for the awkward boob-squeezing torture device!

Mammogram is the best imaging for seeing calcium deposits. It can also find masses and take a peek at the lymph nodes. While many of you have only heard of "the mass," some of you were told that you have calcium in your breast. You might be thinking, What gives? Well, there are a ton of reasons why the breast makes calcium deposits. Not all calcium is concerning. (Thank goodness for all the radiologists out there telling us what is benign calcium and what is worrisome calcium!) But here's one way to understand why cancer makes calcium. First, remember that cancer is a whole lotta bad cookies (cells). These cookies are getting made so fast that they run out of ingredients, or, simply put, the cells outgrow their blood supply and die. The body doesn't like dead cells causing a ruckus, and it builds little calcium walls around these cells (kinda like how some trash requires two trash bags!). Ta-da! A tell-tale clue that there's a problem.

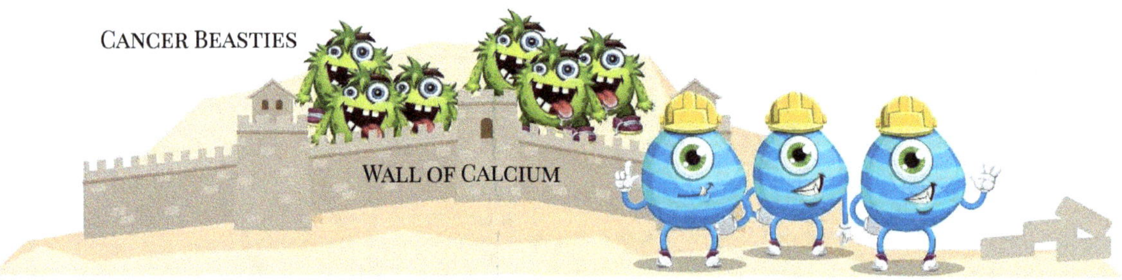

Ultrasound

Ultrasound for the breast is the same thing as a sonogram for pregnancy. It's excellent at finding masses, it's the best imaging for lymph nodes, and it's the easiest way to biopsy things. And, because it's the easiest way to biopsy things, you may be asked to get an additional ultrasound if an MRI or mammogram finds something new in your breast. The radiologists first see if they can find that new mass on ultrasound. If they are able to, they can biopsy it using ultrasound as their guide. Otherwise, you'll be stuck with a mammogram or MRI-guided biopsy. And if you thought an ultrasound-guided biopsy was bad, wait until you need a mammogram or MRI-guided biopsy! Warning: MRI biopsies are darn uncomfortable and technically challenging!

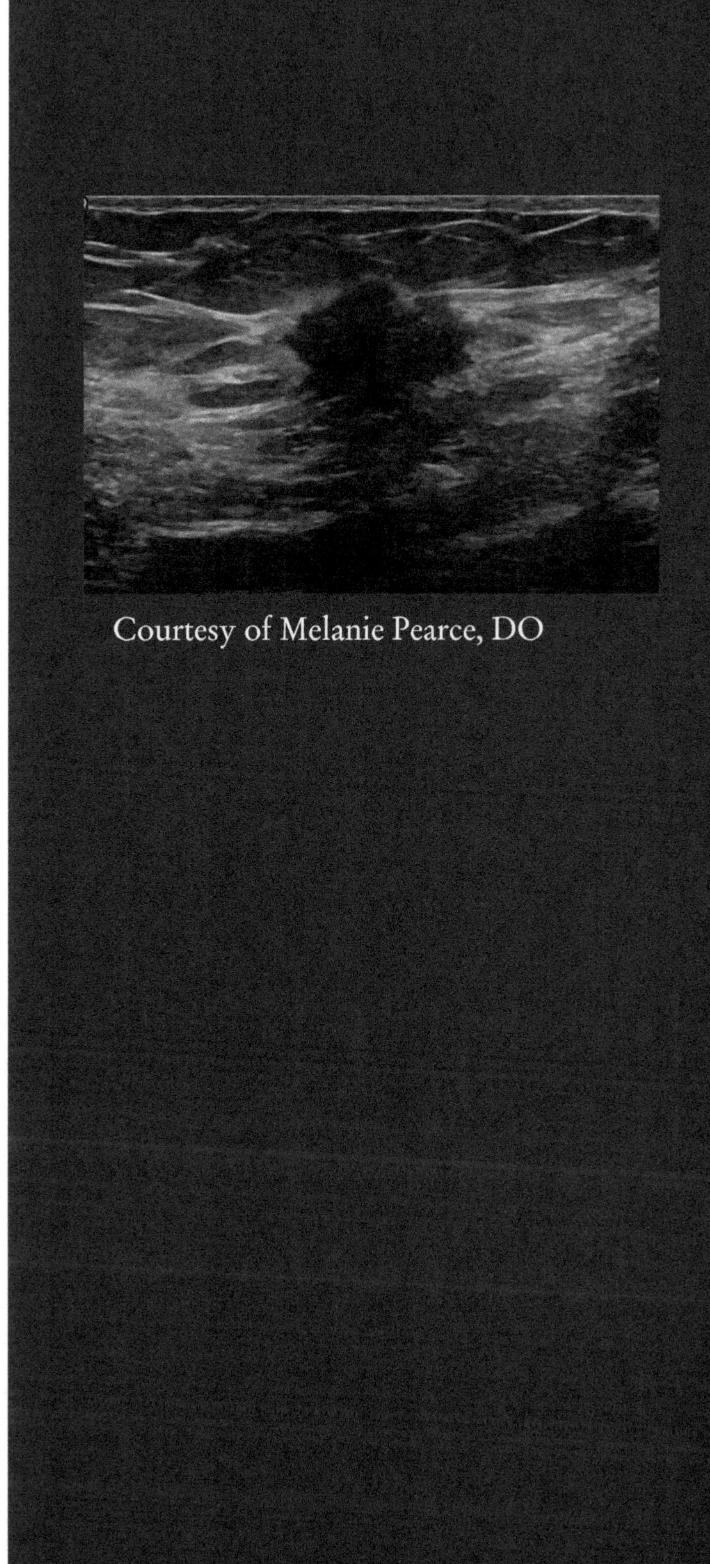

Courtesy of Melanie Pearce, DO

Breast MRI (Magnetic Resonance Imaging)

Super-strong magnets generate these images. MRIs are excellent at finding just about everything in the breast (for better or worse). So, they see everything . . . We want to know it all, right? But the flip side is . . . Crap! They see everything. As such, you may need more biopsies after getting your first one. If you have been offered a breast MRI and you are still trying to decide if MRI is right for you, then make sure you check out a "Detailed and Debated Debrief on MRI" by Dr. Alan Hollingsworth in the Expert Extras Chapter at the end of this book on page 179.

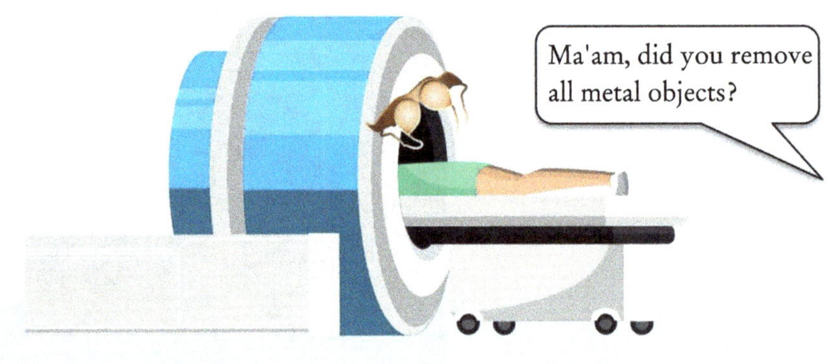

Words from Your Sisters:

You are not alone!

Every woman who has had breast cancer remembers the time in her life when she first heard the words,"You have cancer." It's devastating. It can't be you. You're a mother, wife, busy woman who doesn't have time for this. Well, it was you, and you do have to deal with it. I've been a nurse for thirty-eight years and have taken care of hundreds of cancer patients. I was never a cancer patient. It's something that I "couldn't get" as I have no breast cancer or any cancer history in my family. I've done all the right things. I had children, breastfed them, never took estrogen, ate fairly healthy, exercised when the mood hit me. I always had perfect cancer screening results, never a worry. We moved a few years ago, and I missed my annual mammogram because we were busy. After two years, at age fifty-six, I scheduled the exam and had to go for a repeat, which was a first. I was not worried. When I had the second one, the tech came to get me to see the radiologist, and she asked if I had anyone with me. Well, I knew that wasn't good; something was wrong. The radiologist was very calm and told me I had breast cancer. She said it was quite extensive and that I might need a mastectomy. What? I was in shock. Being a nurse, I had him show me my films. The dead cancer cells leave calcifications that on an X-ray look like white pencil leads. Well, I had lots of them.

Survivor Sister

If you're thinking, "Give me some more info on all this imaging," then read on!

Ultrasound

Here comes a fancy-schmancy word: piezoelectric. This may surprise you, but ultrasound machines use crystals! Yep, ultrasounds work like a bat using echolocation (an ultrasound of the heart is called an echo). The ultrasound probe sends out sound (hence the "sound" part of ultrasound). Some of that sound bounces off our insides and goes right back toward the ultrasound probe while some of the sound waves go straight on through our insides. The sound waves that don't bounce back and the sound waves that do bounce back create an image with the help of some computer wizardry. The sound waves that do bounce back are interpreted by the crystals using the piezoelectric effect. (In this rare case, I do suggest that you turn to Google to find an informative YouTube video if your interest is piqued.) I know, it's crazy, right? Science is amazing!

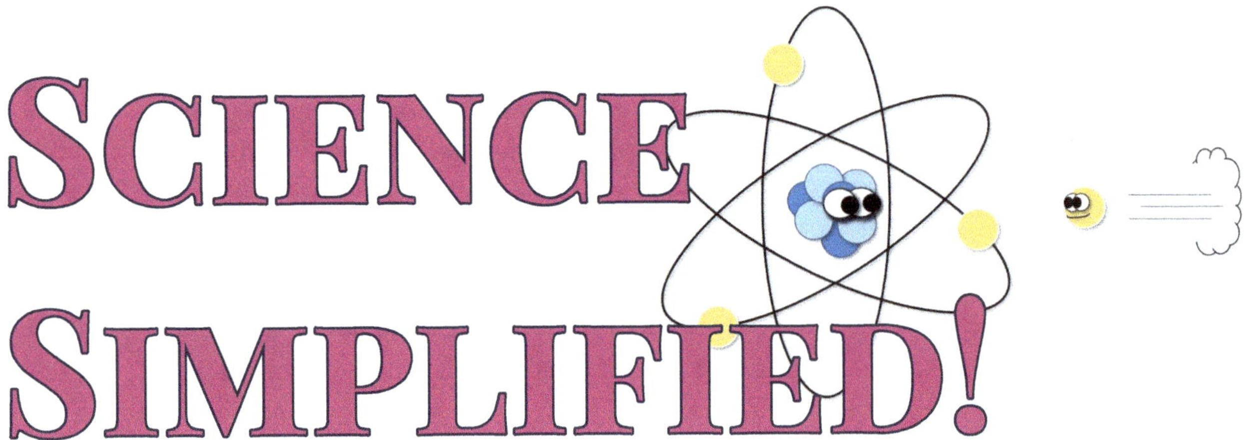

WARNING: PHYSICS AHEAD. PROCEED WITH CAUTION.

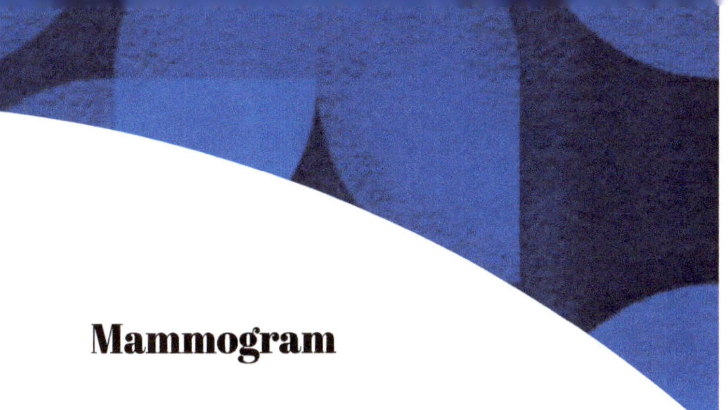

Mammogram

We are going to briefly skim the surface of some pretty amazing science that is way beyond the scope of this book! But here's the gist. X-rays are produced by electrons smashing into atoms. (Atoms are made up of protons, neutrons, and electrons.) If you skipped out on this day in school, think of the smallest particle of matter, the smallest fundamental building block of everything (from our bodies to the stars), and imagine it smashing into the next bigger building block. This is some abstract, teeny-tiny stuff. How tiny, you ask? Well, if all the atoms in your hand were the size of a marble, your hand would be the size of the earth!

The way we get an image is the same way we see our shadows on a sunny day. The sun is representative of the source of the X-rays. Our insides are us, and the image generated is like the shadow we see on the ground. Our bodies stop all the sunlight from reaching the ground, producing one cohesive shadow blob. However, X-rays are definitely different than sunlight. Only the more solid stuff (like the calcium or dense tissue in the breast) can stop the X-rays. So the shadow generated makes an image of only this more solid stuff. Over time, we have gotten pretty sophisticated with X-rays: enter the mammogram in all its forms (2D, digital, and now 3D). Oh, and a CT scan is just a super-fancy 3D version of X-rays. Amazing, right?

MRI

Are you still with me? Let's really get crazy. We've talked electrons and atoms (made up of protons, neutrons, and electrons), but now let's take a closer look at the proton. MRIs are huge magnets (which is why you cannot have one if you have specific devices or prosthetics in your body, and why you cannot wear your favorite jewelry to an MRI party). First, these magnets align all the protons in our bodies (pretend the protons are all like little compass needles). Then comes the radio waves . . . these cause the protons (remember, compass needles) to dance about. When the radio waves stop and those dancing protons realign, they send out their own radio waves that are then interpreted using MRI coils (the information collectors) and some heavy-duty computers. Ta-da! Crazy-cool images, especially of the "soft tissue" (i.e., the non-bone stuff, like breasts).

Sassy Story

Who Decided to X-ray Boobs?

Well, it all started in 1885, when German mechanical engineer and physicist Wilhelm Conrad Röntgen produced and detected "X-radiation." He wasn't quite sure what this new energy was, so he called it X for "unknown." A few experiments later, he realized that this new radiation could see inside people and that these images could be captured on a photographic plate. This was a significant discovery, and for it he received the Nobel Prize in Physics in 1901.

Now, scientists are curious cats, and Dr. Albert Salomon got the bright idea to start taking X-rays of breast specimens *after* mastectomy. He realized that X-rays could see cancers in the breast. (Remember that these were big cancers women could feel in their breasts; there wasn't yet a way to find the small cancers!) He also realized that calcium deposits were in these breast X-rays. However, he didn't make the leap to realizing that calcium could be a sign of cancer. (Let's not hold it against him; we aren't perfect either.) It then took some scientists and doctors quite a few decades to realize the full potential of X-rays in detecting breast cancer in women. Scientific inquiry into the use of mammograms to find cancers that were too small to feel (i.e., as a screening tool) were ongoing throughout the '60s and '70s. Still, it was not until the 1980s that screening mammograms became widespread. And, as we have discussed, the mammogram has made some significant changes since it first came on the scene!

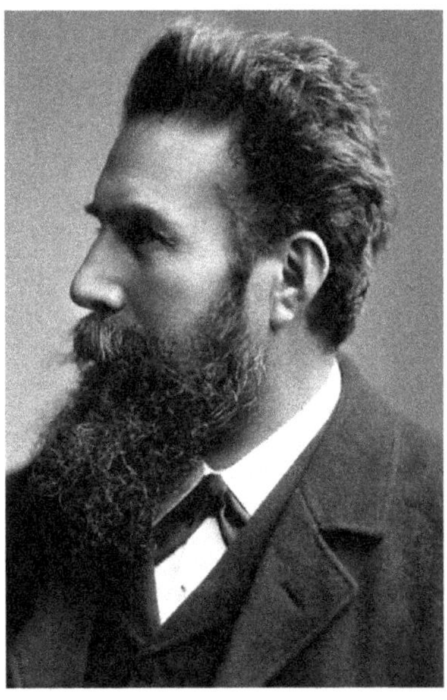

WILHELM RÖNTGEN

Words from your Sisters:

You are not alone!

So, cancer has taken a lot. I wish I never had it. I cried the night before my big surgery, as I would be a different woman for my husband. Fortunately, he loves me the way I am! Thank goodness! I have my friends and my cancer friends. The cancer friends are the ones you can talk to about your breast concerns or show them your nipple tattoo, and they get excited. My other friends wouldn't know how to take that. You have to always have goals and keep reaching them. I just became a grandmother for the first time, and that's something worth being around for!

Survivor Sister

FAQS:

Frequently Asked Questions

Q. Did all those mammograms cause my cancer? Doesn't radiation cause cancer?

A. All right, ladies. If you are trying to connect the dots and this idea popped into your head, then track it down and push it out! Mammograms have decreased breast cancer mortality (death) by upwards of 40 percent. It is the single most effective intervention to improve a woman's chance of surviving breast cancer!

Q. How much radiation is in a mammogram?

A. A 2D mammogram has the same amount of radiation exposure as about six weeks of living on planet earth. (Yes! We are all exposed to radiation every day, all day.) The newer 3D mammograms have slightly more radiation than this. But the bottom line is this: Don't blame your past diligence in getting annual mammograms for the creation of your cancer. And certainly don't skip mammograms for fear of radiation!

Q. How many cancers does a mammogram miss (i.e., was this sucker there last year?)?

A. Well, first off, there's 2D plain film mammograms, digital mammograms, and 3D mammograms. Almost everywhere you go nowadays, you will at least get a digital mammogram. Digital means that it is on the computer screen instead of those big floppy printed images that get hung on a lightbox on the wall. Many places are now able to offer 3D or tomosynthesis imaging. I say this because there are a couple of ways to answer this question, and I don't want you to get the wrong idea.

The simple answer is: this is a moving target. Up to 20 percent of women without breast symptoms (masses, nipple discharge, etc.) will get a mammogram and be told there is no cancer in her breasts when, in fact, there is (some studies report even higher numbers with increased breast density). Ladies, nothing is perfect! And this doesn't mean that the radiologist messed up; it just means that the tool they use isn't perfect. In contrast, a breast MRI only misses about 1 percent of breast cancers. And in case you are thinking, Breast MRI for everyone! Ditch the mammogram! Wait, wait, and wait. There is a trade-off to breast MRI. Remember, breast MRI finds everything, which can lead to more unnecessary biopsies and the associated stress of benign biopsies. And in case you're still thinking, "well, that's small beans to find cancer!" It's really not that simple. You also need to factor in time, money, the risks of more unnecessary procedures, and the potential risks of the IV dye that must be administered with MRI. Alas, nothing is truly perfect. However, because breast MRI has a leg up on finding cancers, women at high risk of developing cancer get screening breast MRIs every year in addition to a screening mammogram. When I say high risk, I mean that they are at twice the average woman's risk.

Words from Your Sisters:

You are not alone!

Each woman has a different journey. I thought when you had breast cancer, it was treated, it was all the same. Oh no. Anyone diagnosed has a different path. It's all in the details.

Survivor Sister

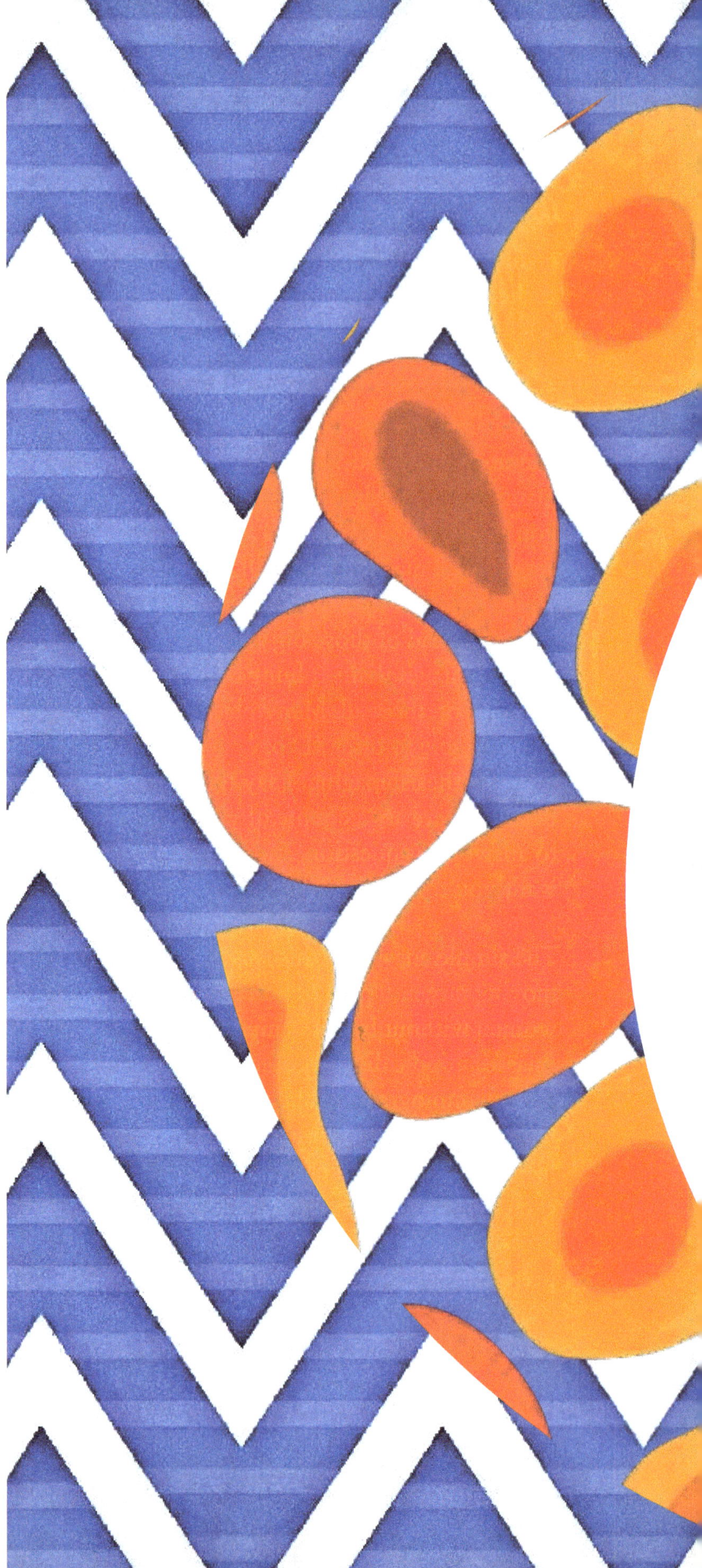

Pathology

Ouch! Someone Poked Me!

Biopsies are far from fun (to put it mildly). But, we need them. You have already taken this step, otherwise, we wouldn't be here. So let's not relive that experience.

Unlike your radiology reports, the pathologists put the "bottom line" synoptic report at the very top. You usually only need to read the first page to get the diagnosis and the critical information that you need.

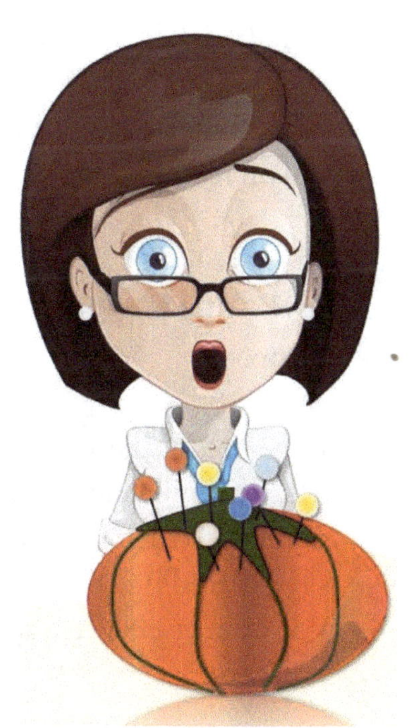

First, let's back up and recall: "What is cancer?"

Go back to the family recipe written in your grandmother's handwriting. Every day our bodies are making new cells using this recipe, and every new batch of cookies comes from a newly copied recipe. Grandma's cursive can be tricky, mistakes are made, and things get downright wacky when you copy over and over and over. We have a lot of checks and balances in place to prevent errors (like, "Hey, Mom, what does this say?"), but as mistakes accumulate, that once-great recipe can turn into a disaster. The same thing can happen in our bodies. The cells that are supposed to be those wonderful, ooey-gooey, chocolate-chip oatmeal cookies (normal cells) slowly morph into salty cardboard (cancer). Cancer is just the summation of mistakes made in the written recipe. Then, one day you aren't making breast cells; instead, you're making cancer cells. And those copied recipes continue to be copied, making even more mistakes. This means that not every batch of cookies in that clump of cancer is made from the same recipe. They are an amalgam of all the recipes along the way. There are some cookie batches with too much salt, and there are some cookies batches where the baking soda was left out. So, cancer is not all from the same recipe (the cells are not, strictly speaking, clones). This is why some women, for example, have cancers that are not 100 percent positive for estrogen receptors. If you look closely at your pathology report, you may find that your "estrogen-positive" cancer is only 40 percent or 60 percent estrogen positive. It's a mixed bag! If your first thought was, Receptors? have no fear. By the end of this chapter, you'll be a receptor aficionado!

There are many different things that a pathology report could say that ultimately means "cancer." We will cover the basics here. But if you have a zebra (the medical community's term for rare) type of cancer, you might not find it here. No fear! Your doc will explain it at your visit.

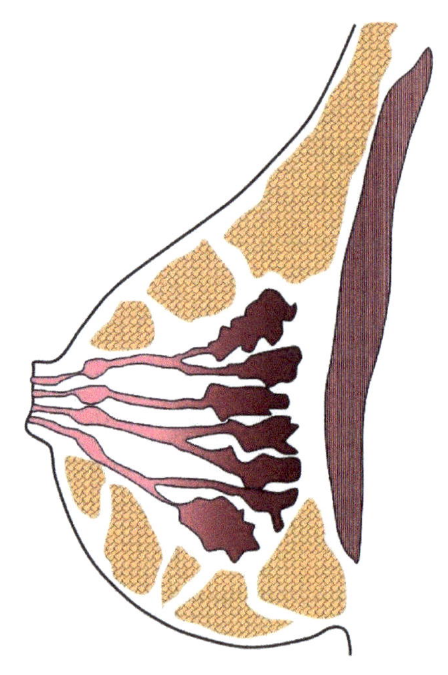

Ductal and Lobular Carcinoma (Cancer)

In the breast, there are lobules that make the milk and ducts that carry that milk out to the nipple when a woman is breastfeeding. The most common type of breast cancer (accounting for 80 to 85 percent of all breast cancers) arises from the ducts. Ducts are basically the plumbing of the breast. They are the pipes that carry the milk from the lobules (where the milk is made) to the nipple. Under a microscope, they look just like a pipe—hollow on the inside with a regular appearing wall. However, unlike pipes, these lady pipes are made of cells (the cookies). And it's when these cells start getting made from a bum recipe that cancer is formed. Sometimes when these cells start growing, they multiply inside the pipe, filling up the center of the duct (otherwise referred to as a lumen). Ultimately, they "clog" the duct with cancer cells. Voilà, that's the definition of a ductal (arises from the duct cells) carcinoma (cancer) in situ (inside the duct), which is abbreviated as DCIS and is considered a "noninvasive breast cancer." This is Stage 0 breast cancer, and it is not supposed to spread outside of the breast.

Sometimes, however, the cells go so haywire that they start making travel plans. They breach the walls of the pipe and run amok in the tissue outside of the duct.

This is known as invasive ductal carcinoma (IDC)

Invasive = invade the tissue outside the duct

Ductal = arising from the ducts

Carcinoma = cancer

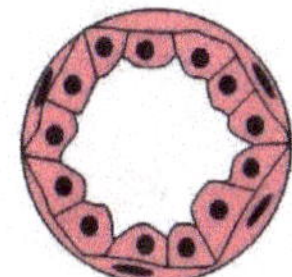

Normal Duct

Looks like a water pipe with a hollow center and regular appearing walls.

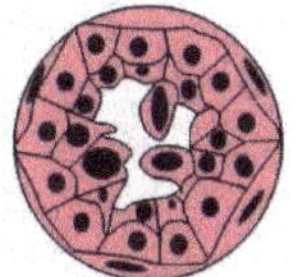

DCIS

Also referred to as "non-invasive cancer." Looks like a clogged pipe.

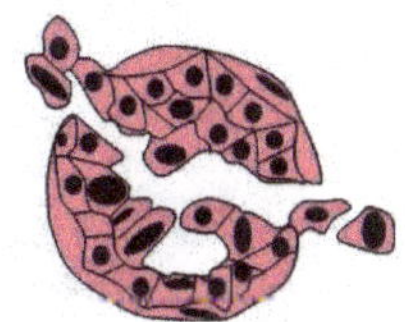

Invasive Cancer

Looks like a broken pipe with cells spilling into the nearby fatty tissue of the breast.

The next most common type of cancer arises from the lobules (or milk maker sacs); these account for about 10 to 15 percent of the breast cancers diagnosed every year. This is called invasive lobular carcinoma (ILC). It's the same idea as invasive ductal cancer. The exception is that lobular carcinoma in situ (LCIS) is not itself considered cancer (yes, confusing). Why is it different? Well, there is some significant debate in the literature (which is jargon for "we aren't sure"). The bottom line is that, at the very least, LCIS places a woman at increased risk of breast cancer (in both breasts); this is called a high-risk lesion. And, at the worst, it could become invasive cancer (enter multi-decade debate). Anyway, invasive lobular carcinoma (ILC) is treated in the same way that invasive ductal carcinoma is; it just arises from another structure (think of them like evil cousins). Also, realize that ILC is sneaky. Instead of forming nests of cells that, in turn, form discrete masses, ILC forms strands of abnormal cells in and among otherwise normal tissue. This means that the overall size can be underestimated on imaging. Imaging sees big stuff; it does not see cells. Sneaky? Yes! But treatable? Yes!

The next thing you will see on your pathology report is the "grade." You may be thinking, I am going to get graded now? Geeze! No, you can relax. The grade is simply a score the pathologist gives the cancer cells to communicate how normal or abnormal the cells are.

THE GRADE IS NOT THE SAME AS YOUR STAGE!

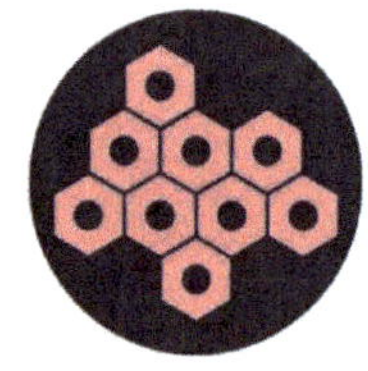

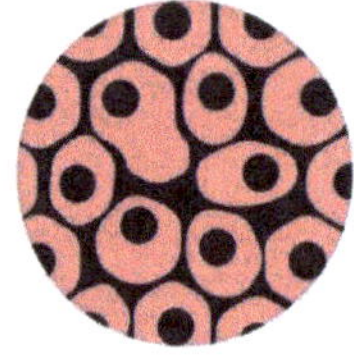

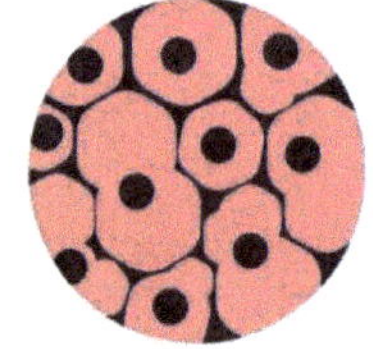

Grade 1
"These cells look pretty normal, but they are not where they are supposed to be!"

Grade 2
"These cells aren't normal, but . . . they also don't look too bad."

Grade 3
Something akin to, "Is that even a breast cell?"

And Finally, We Get to Receptors!

These little suckers will play a huge role in determining what treatments you do or don't get and may help to decide the order of those treatments!

So, what on earth is a receptor? Well, ladies, let's imagine the breast cancer cell is a house, and the receptors are the satellite dishes or TV antennae on the roof. These receptors or satellite dishes are there to receive signals being broadcast by the body just like the satellite dishes on the roof receive signals. They give those signals to the house or breast cancer cell.

Now some breast cancers are like that "interesting" house on the street with three satellite dishes and five TV antennae. (What on earth is going on there?) This means that they have put up a whole bunch of receptors. The good news about having a ton of receptors? We can target an attack of just the cells with those receptors—BOOM!

There are three receptors that we look for in breast cancer. (You can have all three receptors, no receptors, or any combination of these receptors.):

Estrogen Receptor (ER)

Progesterone Receptor (PR)

HER2-neu Receptor

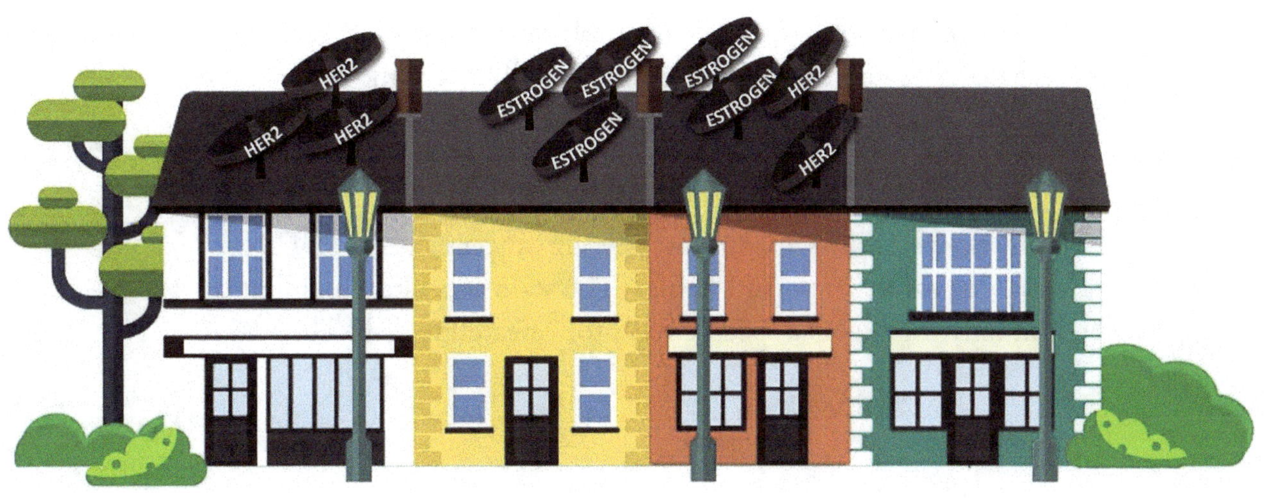

ER-, PR-, HER2+	ER+, PR- HER2-	ER+, PR-, HER2+	ER-, PR-, HER2-

Estrogen and progesterone are hormone receptors. This means that any time one of those cancer cells sees estrogen or progesterone, they are getting the signal to grow (later, we will discuss our strategy to cut this signal off). Now, remember that your cancer is not a clone of one cancer cell; cancer is heterogeneous (this is the fancy word for "mixed bag"). So, while the first question is "Are there estrogen and progesterone receptors present?" the second question is, "What percentage of cancer cells have those receptors?" Enter the awesome pathologists who tell us all this information. When you talk to your doc about this, you may hear them say that your cancer is "strongly positive" or "weakly positive," which reflects the percentage of cells with too many satellite dishes. Since they are a target for treatment, the more the better!

The third type of receptor that we look for in breast cancer is not a hormone receptor. The HER2-neu receptor is another type of satellite dish on the roof that some smart scientists found in about 30 percent of breast cancers. Then, some more smart scientists invented medications to specifically attack cells with only those receptors. (A targeted attack on cancer cells? Yes! Kapow!)

Now, some of you are looking at this list and thinking, What about me? All three of my receptors are all negative. If this is the case, you have a "triple-negative" breast cancer. So if your breast cancer houses aren't gaudy with satellite dishes, this means that you aren't a candidate for estrogen-blocking meds or HER2-targeted therapy. But have no fear. We still have some cards up our sleeves, chicka, for better or worse. Spoiler alert: it's chemo . . . more on this later.

How do we know what receptors your cancer cells have? The pathologists have special "stains." The stain acts like a highlighter that only highlights a specific receptor or satellite dish. The estrogen receptor stain highlights only the estrogen receptors. It leaves the rest of the cells on the slide mostly blank. The progesterone receptor stain highlights only the progesterone receptors. It leaves the rest of the cells on the slide mostly blank. The pathologist will let us know how many satellite dishes are on each house (intensity) and what percentage of houses have satellite dishes (percentage).

The HER2 receptor has its own rules. The initial HER2 receptor stain highlights only the receptors for HER2 and leaves the rest of the cells, again, mostly blank. Unfortunately, sometimes this initial stain is "equivocal" or "I dunno?" In this case, a special test is performed to confirm the receptor status; this is usually called a FISH or DISH test. Either way, your pathologist will tell your clinical docs if you are positive or negative for each receptor!

I can hear the questions forming in your mind:

"What's my stage, doc?"
"What are my odds"?
"Am I going to live?"

The bottom line is, no one can tell you yes, no, or your exact survival rate. We could all get hit by a bus tomorrow, right? I know—blah, blah, blah. Anyway, the stage of breast cancer was once determined by TNM, which represents three things: the size of the Tumor in the breast (T), the presence of cancer in the lymph Nodes (N), and the presence of cancer in some other part of the body (M for Metastasis).

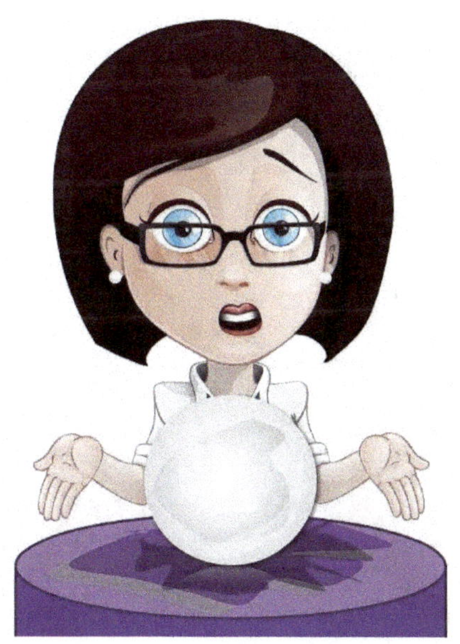

However, in 2018 this was revised to consider some other key factors. Also, an important asterisk, this new staging system also assumes that you're going to finish all the recommended therapy! Now, it's not just TNM. We add the grade and all three receptors into the mix (and for some women, an additional factor, their Oncotype Dx score®, will be added in—more on this later). That's around seven or eight variables, a massive algorithm. But don't worry, there are phone apps and online calculators.

But even with these improvements, you need to realize that each stage has some hugely different people factors and types of cancers all lumped together. For example, these two cancers are in the same stage: Stage IB.

> 2.1cm ER/PR+ HER2 - grade 1 cancer without cancer in the lymph nodes
>
> 4.9cm ER/PR+ HER2 + grade 3 cancer with lymph node metastasis (cancer in the lymph nodes under the arm)

So, while stage is much talked about, it is really more suited for dealing with studies of populations than acting as a crystal ball for individuals. Please don't hang your hat on some percentage tied to your stage. Keep living life, one moment at a time, and forget about labeling your life according to a percentage.

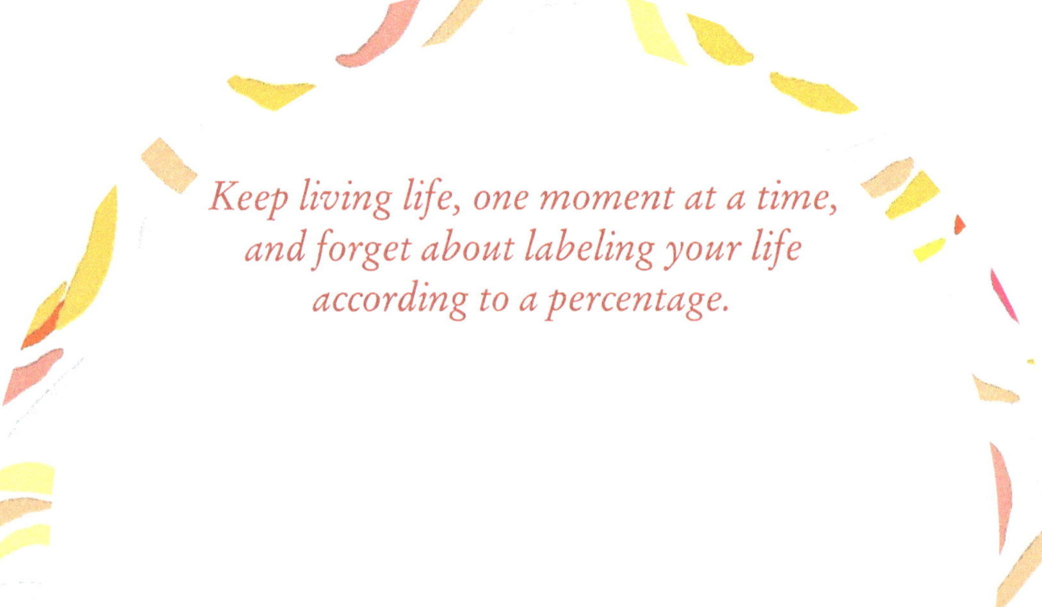

Sampling Error

Yay! My biopsy was benign . . .

All right, so you got squished and poked. But anytime a biopsy is performed, it's important to understand the limitation of this poking and prodding! And for that, let's bring in the analogy!

Imagine a beautiful field of wildflowers on a perfect, sunny day. It's 75 degrees with a slight breeze. Go ahead and close your eyes, take a nice deep breath, hold for the count of five, and exhale. Repeat three times. Okay, now for real. Let's get back to business. You are still looking at a beautiful field of wildflowers of all different colors. Imagine you pick four flowers and bring them home. What colors are they? Let's say they are all purple.

Now, if you brought that bouquet to your best gal pal and asked her what color the field of wildflowers is? She might incorrectly assume that the whole field consists of purple wildflowers. Buzz! Wrong, sister! You took a "sample" of flowers; you didn't pick the whole field! Your small sample doesn't reflect the whole field.

Now apply this to cancer. Let's say someone biopsied an area in the breast and said, "It's DCIS." Hurrah! No invasive cancer here, girlfriend! Or let's say an abnormal lymph node is biopsied and someone said, "No cancer in the lymph nodes." Wait! That is just like the purple bouquet. Purple being DCIS or a benign biopsy. Unfortunately, there can be that pesky old "sampling error." There can be yellow flowers (invasive cancer) in there too! We just didn't pick those flowers with our limited sample.

If you had a biopsy of a lymph node or some other area of concern in the breast and it was benign, or if you have a diagnosis of DCIS, there's not a 100 percent guarantee that there's no invasive cancer. Period. So how do we solve this? Let's mow the field and pick all those flowers!

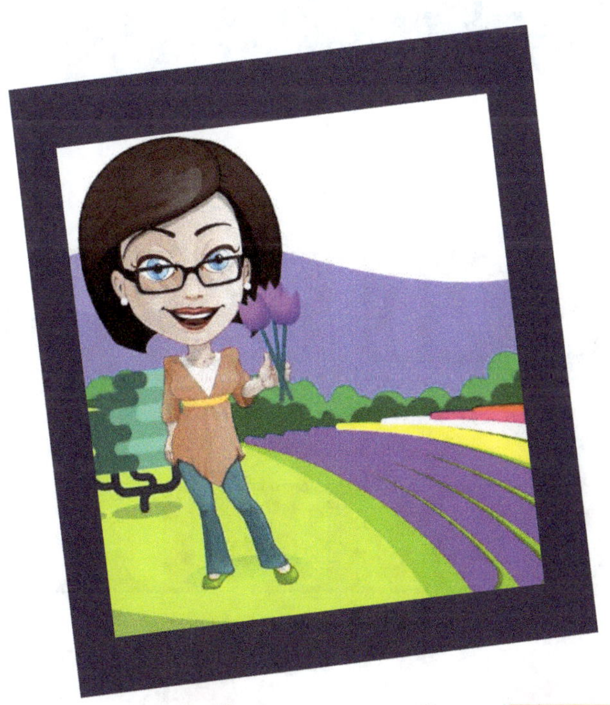

This section is better told in picture format. Feast your eyes on all the pretty colors . . . those cells are the building blocks of these amazing bodies we all inhabit! And the rest of the photos are the bad cookies. Ick!

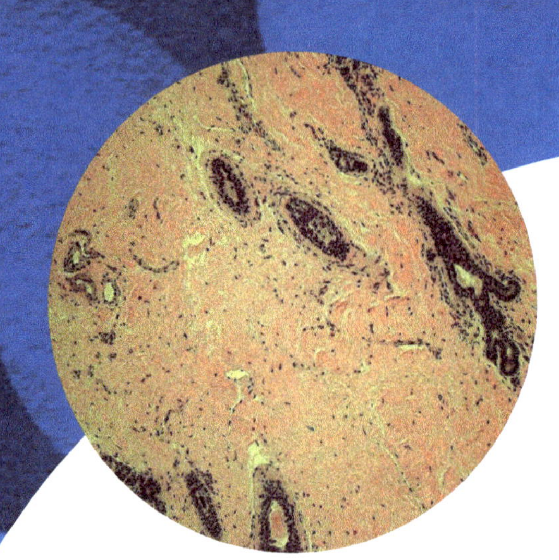

Normal Breast

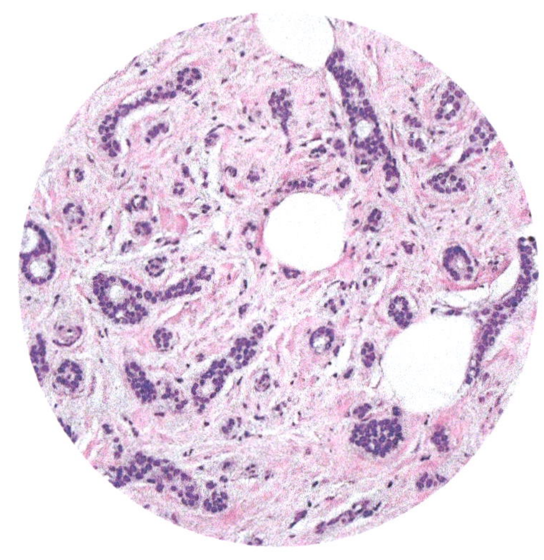

Invasive Ductal Carcinoma (IDC)

SCIENCE SIMPLIFIED!

Invasive Lobular Carcinoma (ILC)

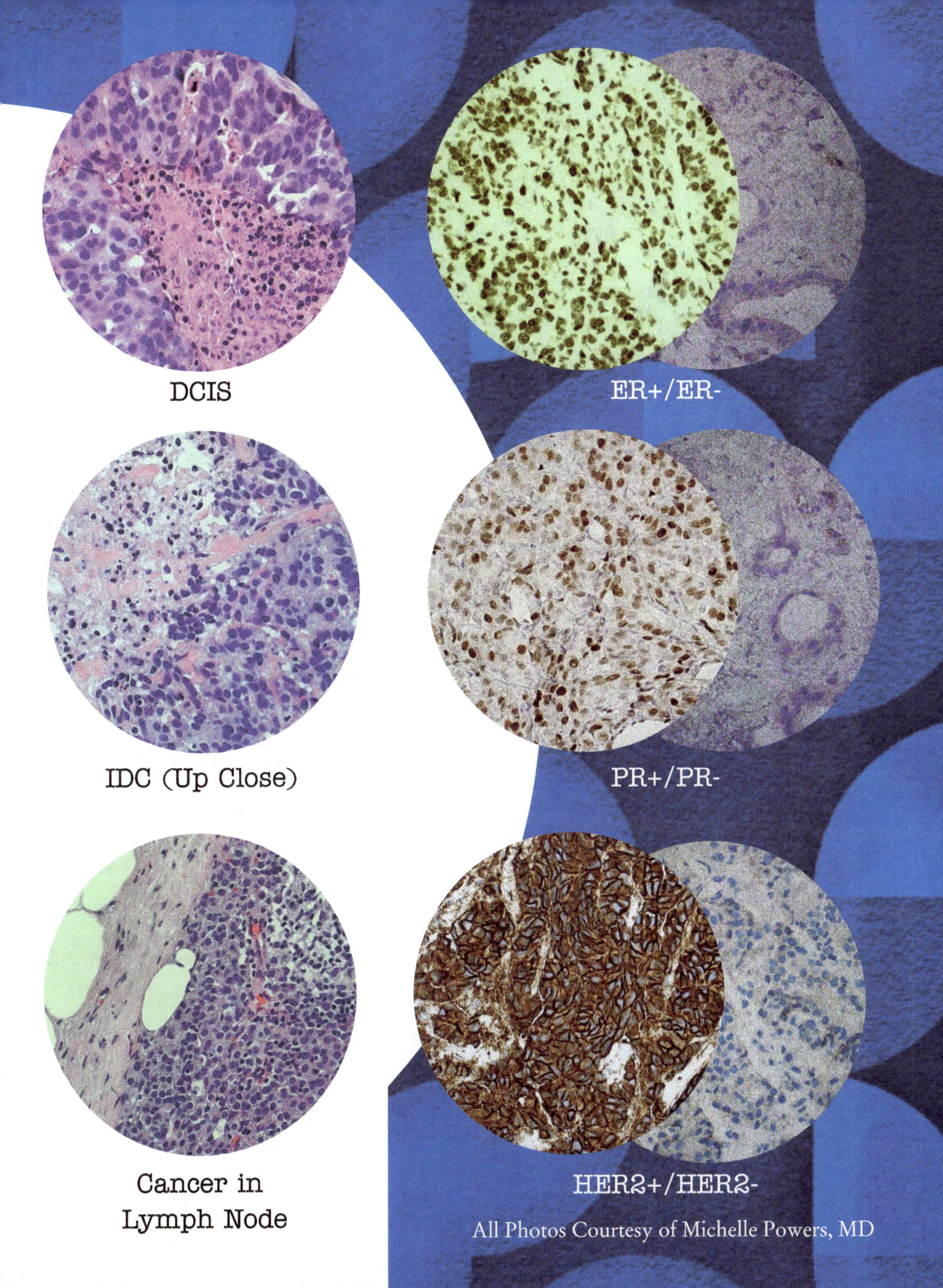

All Photos Courtesy of Michelle Powers, MD

Sassy Story

People wandered around for a really long time not realizing we are made up of many tiny cells. This is knowledge that we take for granted nowadays. But the first time someone was able to see a single cell was Robert Hooke in 1665 after he invented the microscope. And this guy came up with the word "cell" because he thought that the plant cell he was looking at reminded him of a monk's living quarters. Now, looking at cells under the microscope can be a little bland. Enter special stains and all the pretty colors. We use these to help our eyes discern details and highlight receptors. Yep! Those estrogen, progesterone, and HER2 receptors don't just hang neon signs on the cell's storefront! We have to go looking for them.

The most commonly used stain, the "H&E" stain, was first pioneered in 1876 by Mr. A. Wissowzky. It helps the pathologist see the details of the cells more clearly so that they can tell us, "This is cancer" and "This is a grade 3 cancer." But, truth be told, the world of pathology is filled with many, many, many stains, and stains help us arrive at the diagnosis listed on your pathology report.

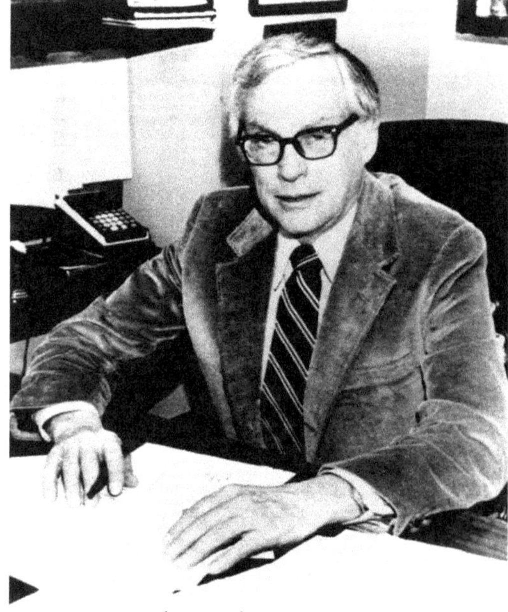

Elwood V. Jensen
General Motors Cancer Research Foundation

Estrogen receptors were discovered in 1958 by Elwood V. Jensen in Chicago; he is considered by some to be the father of hormone receptors. The progesterone receptor was then found in the 1970s. And finally, the Her2-neu receptor was initially found in rat studies in 1984.

FAQS:

Frequently Asked Questions

Q. Can the cancer be spread through my breast by the biopsy needle?

A. This is called "seeding" in the medical field. Seeding is the idea that the biopsy needle drags some of the cancer cells through the tissue on its way out. We do not typically worry about breast cancer cells spreading at the time of biopsy (although there are some types of cancer where we certainly do worry about this). Luckily, this has been studied. The conclusion is that breast biopsy is safe because the cancer cells left in the wake of the needle tract are largely nonviable (meaning they die). Now, that doesn't mean that there aren't some accounts of local recurrence (cancer coming back in the breast) that could be due to this phenomenon. But remember that the tract is typically treated with radiation in the case of breast conservation. And, depending on the location of the cancer, the tract is commonly removed at the time of mastectomy. We have more important things to focus on. The biopsy opens the door to your complete treatment plan. Let's move on!

Q. There "wasn't enough tissue" obtained at my first biopsy, and now I don't know what my receptors are. What gives?

A. Yes, this can happen. Remember that special stains are done to help the pathologist tell us what, if any, receptors are there. And each of these stains needs its own teeny-tiny sliver of tissue (you only get one stain per slide). So, if they run out of cancer tissue to test, you are without this information. Now, unless you have some itty-bitty tiny cancer that is completely removed at the time of the biopsy, then the remainder of the tumor removed at the time of surgery will give us this information. I know . . . the suspense, right?

Words from Your Sisters:

You are not alone!

Life gives you challenges, and you just have to meet them head-on and survive! One thing that is so important about the cancer journey is remembering that you will live your life for hopefully many, many years. We don't want to be disfigured from a quick decision at the beginning. It needs to be the decision that you can live with ten years and twenty years from now.

Survivor Sister

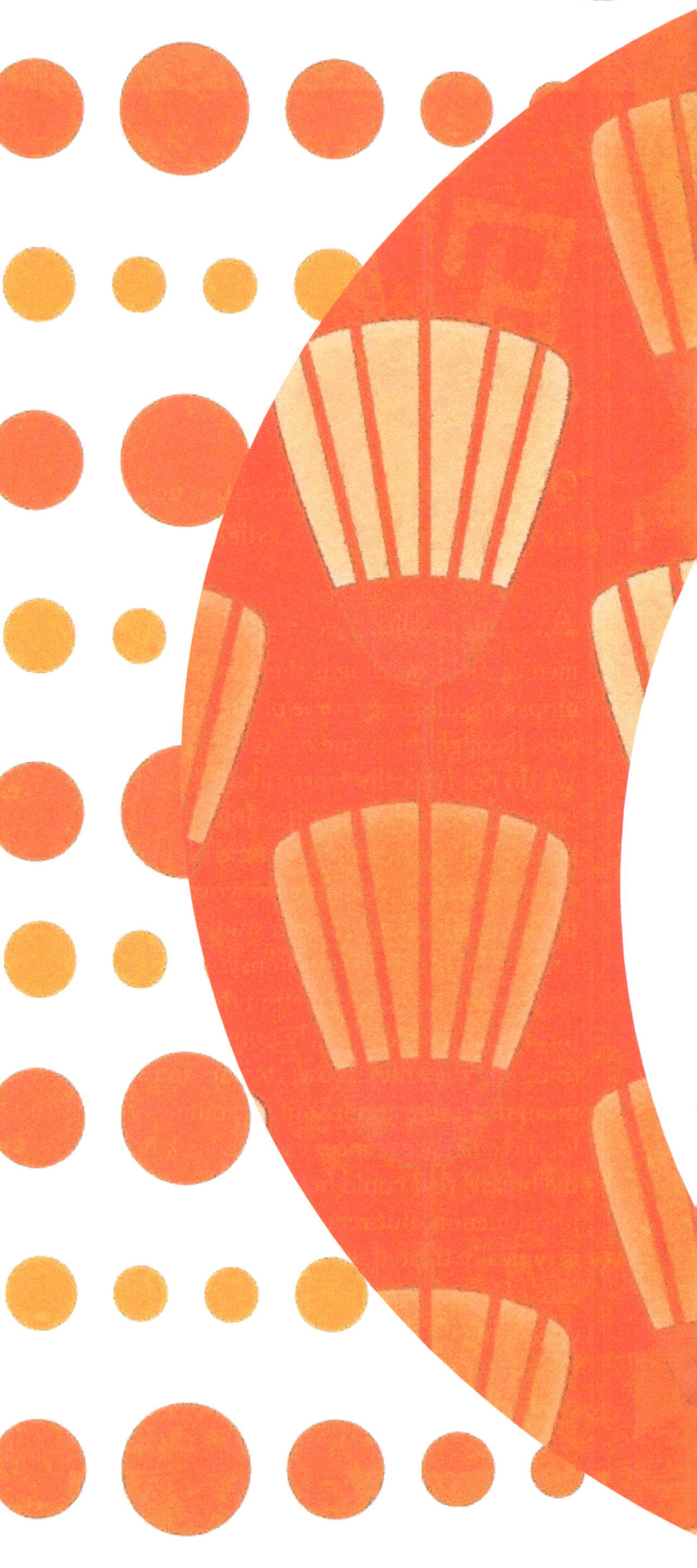

Surgery

Am I Going to Lose My Breasts?

All right, sweet pea. Someone told you there's a mass, or calcifications, or architectural distortion (whatever that means), and now you want that thing gone yesterday, or maybe even last year. Five-alarm anxiety is hitting you, and you want that "crab" out. (Side factoid: the Greek word for "crab" is the root of the word *cancer*.)

There's no "one size fits all" rule here. You need a surgeon you trust to help you navigate these waters, sailor! Surgical management for breast cancer can and should be personalized to you. No sassy book will be able to make this decision for you, but let me offer some ground rules so that you come to the table with an essential toolkit to help you build your treatment plan. Breast cancer is not as simple as some other cancers. There are a fair number (if not most) of cancers where the surgeon simply tells you what the treatment is—no choices, no discussion, she just tells you the "what's what." Breast cancer is usually not so simple. There are options for most ladies, and choosing the right one for you can be tough!

Let's start with the basics. What are the goals of surgery? Duh . . . remove the cancer, all of the cancer, put it in a bucket, and say, "See you later, you life-disrupting piece of $#*%." (Oops, I'm getting carried away. Deep breaths . . . moving on!). But really, a surgeon can only offer surgery if they think that they can remove all the cancer. Because who wants to go through the pain and recovery of surgery and still have cancer left in their body? So, the first real question to ask is:

"Am I a candidate for surgery?"

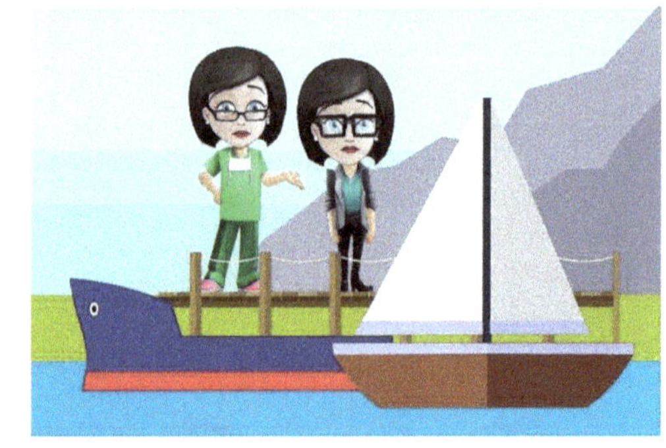

Surgeon: "*Both boats will get you there...*"
Patient: "*But I don't want a boat!*"

This is a question for the experts to figure out! They, in turn, ask the questions like:

1. Has the cancer spread to another part of the body? (Did any of these cells jump on the lymphatic expressway and get off somewhere they are not supposed to be? This is also known as metastasis.)

2. Is it locally aggressive? (Is this cancer trying to worm its way into my chest wall or out through my skin?) Or is it an inflammatory breast cancer (in which case you need chemotherapy first)?

3. Finally, for all you lovely ladies that have lived long, fierce lives and now have the battle scars to prove it (think heart disease, lung disease, maybe another ongoing cancer), we need to ask if surgery is too risky. If so, not to fear, surgery is not the only tool in our toolbox! See the "risks vs. benefits section" on the next page.

So, you've determined that you are a candidate for surgery, the next question most women ask is, "Do I need a mastectomy?" (Mastectomy is the removal of the whole breast.) There is another option here: lumpectomy (aka partial mastectomy). This is the removal of part of the breast (and we will get to that next), but not everyone is a candidate for lumpectomy. So, let's see if there is any medical or anatomical reason you might need a mastectomy before we go and muddy the waters with the pros and cons of each. In other words, size does matter.

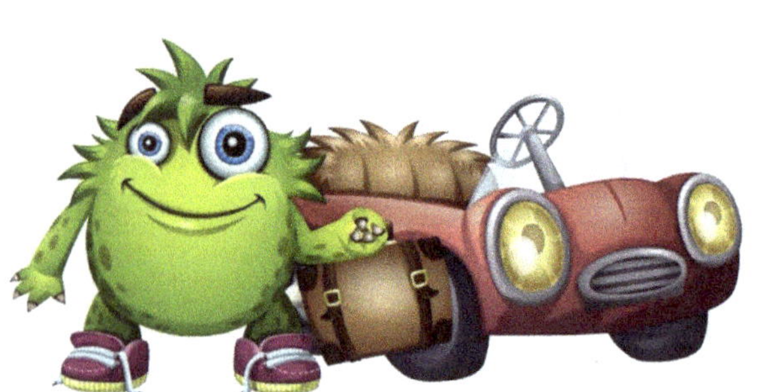

Risks vs. Benefits

Throughout this book, you will be presented with many possible treatment options. Each of these has associated risks; some risks are itty-bitty, teeny-tiny, and some are life-threatening. How risky each treatment is will be different for everyone. Why? Because everyone is coming to the table with different backgrounds (age, health issues, goals). So let's put risk on one side of the scale.

On the other side of the scale are the benefits. Again, some benefits are small, and some are lifesaving. Each therapy option, again, will be different for each person.

Risks and benefits. Risks and benefits . . .

For example, let's take surgery. The benefits of surgery are easy: remove the cancer. The risks of surgery are different for everyone. A thirty-five-year-old marathon runner will sail through the risks of surgery and anesthesia and has another fifty or more years to live; the benefits clearly outweigh the risks. However, a ninety-five-year-old with advanced heart and lung disease who gets chest pain moving from her wheelchair to the bed at night is going to be lucky to survive even a small procedure. The risks are prohibitively higher. The potential benefit of surgery will be lost entirely if this lovely lady dies from surgery or anesthesia complications.

This spectrum of risks and benefits is evaluated by each doctor you see. Each therapy is tailored to you, be it surgery, radiation, chemotherapy, anti-estrogen therapy, etc.

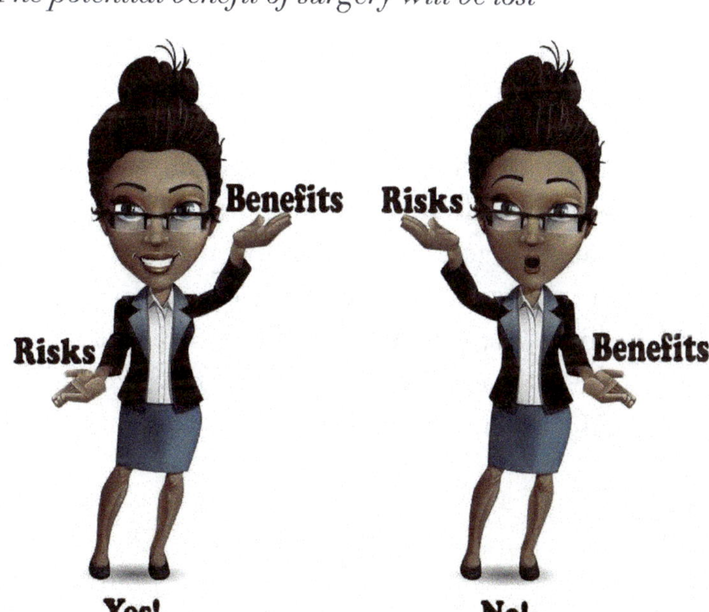

You may need a mastectomy if you have:

1. Big 'Ole Cancer

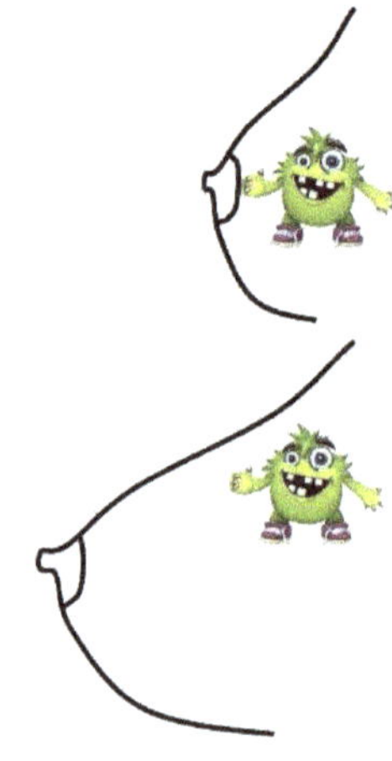

It's not the size of the cancer. It's not the size of the breast. It's the size of the cancer in relation to the size of the breast. Huh? What on earth are we talking about here? Well, let's take a cancer the size of a ping-pong ball (4 cm: yes, doctors usually talk in terms of centimeters, millimeters, and grams). Now, if we have a ping-pong-ball-sized cancer in a woman with an AA cup breast, sorry girlfriend, but that is her whole breast. There's no way to take that entire cancer out with a healthy rim of tissue and leave her with anything that resembles a breast. Conversely, if we take that same ping-pong-ball-sized cancer and put it in an F cup breast, that endowed lady (with a sore back from carrying around those heavy breasts) is not going to miss the ping-pong-ball-sized cancer. In fact, she may want to go for a "two-for-one" deal and have a breast reduction at the same time as her cancer surgery. (Yes, there can be some silver linings here!)

Another idea to keep in mind is, "Can we shrink the cancer and tip the scales back toward lumpectomy?" Possibly! If you are pretty sure lumpectomy is for you, ask your doctor about the options. But remember, the answer might end up being no.

2. Multifocal Cancer

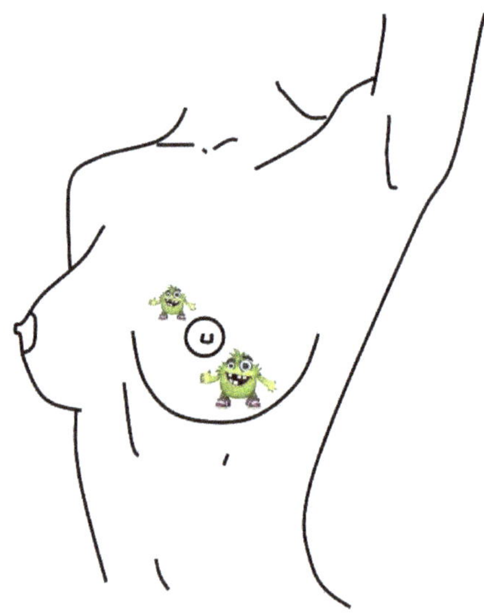

You have more than one cancer in your breast. We generally don't swiss cheese those puppies out. And geez, that breast has already made two or more cancers! Fool me once . . . Now, like all things, there are rules, and there are reasons to break the rules. Enter personalized care and a discussion with your doctor!

Genetic Variants

"Did my genes put me at an increased risk of cancer?"

So, you got tested? Make sure your test says "pathogenic" or "deleterious" before you start making grand plans. Similar to the BI-RADS scoring system, we have a scoring system for genetics too! Five levels, to be exact: normal, benign variant, variant of uncertain significance, likely pathogenic (or deleterious) variant, and pathogenic variant. Keep in mind that different companies use slightly different language. There are plenty of people who test positive for "variants of uncertain/unknown significance," abbreviated as "VUS." VUS means that the test found a difference. Translated, it means, "That lady has something about her gene that is different from most people's genes. But, we don't know if that difference matters." Is it like the difference between you and me, or is it a potential bad actor? These VUS could someday become something considered a pathogenic variant. Or they could prove to be completely normal and stop being reported at all. So, the recommendation is to disregard them and not take any specific clinical action because of them. *See the genetics chapter on page 156 for more info!*

3. Genetic Mutation Carrier

If this is the only box you check in this section, this is not a must. It's your body. Every year plenty of BRCA 1 and BRCA 2 pathogenic genetic variant carriers undergo lumpectomies. For those who have no idea what a BRCA gene is, BRCA 1 and BRCA 2 genes are the most well-known genes that cause breast cancer. However, some studies suggest that more aggressive surgical management (even bilateral mastectomy) improves these ladies' overall survival. That means that genetic mutation carriers live longer if they have their breast removed.

Note: There are plenty of other mutations that have been linked to breast cancer. And the recommendations on what to do for these lovely ladies are always being updated. Instead of putting some quick-to-expire specifics on these things, consult your genetic counselor!

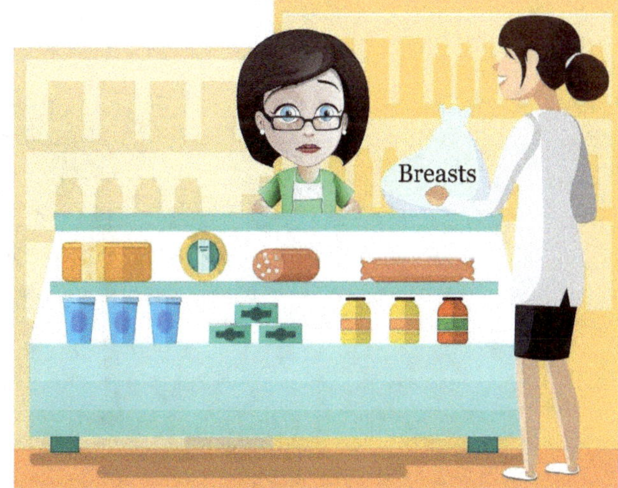

Patient: "*I would like to return these, they are trying to kill me!*

4. Medical Condition That May Preclude Radiation

Lumpectomy equals radiation . . . period. Cough, cough . . . with those few exceptions. (I am looking at you ladies over seventy years of age and for whom the stars align.) For the rest of us, the rate of cancer recurrence after lumpectomy without radiation is as high as 30 to 40 percent. With radiation, this plummets to as low as 5 to 15 percent (remember that the average woman on this earth has a 12.5 percent lifetime risk). So, if you cannot have radiation or will not have radiation, you should not consider a lumpectomy. If you have a prior history of radiation to the chest, specific genetic mutations (p53 gene mutation), or some medical conditions (most of which involve skin and soft tissue disorders), then radiation may not be for you. And if radiation is not for you, then in general, lumpectomy is not for you. However, when in doubt, review this with your radiation oncologist.

If you have read through this list and you *aren't* thinking, "I need a mastectomy," let's talk about your options. Should you get a mastectomy anyway?

If you are one of the many ladies given the option to choose either lumpectomy or mastectomy, why would you choose mastectomy? Here is where it comes down to some very personal decisions, and many women fall into one of two camps. Unfortunately, for some, this is going to be one hell of a hard decision because—shoot—"I just don't know!"

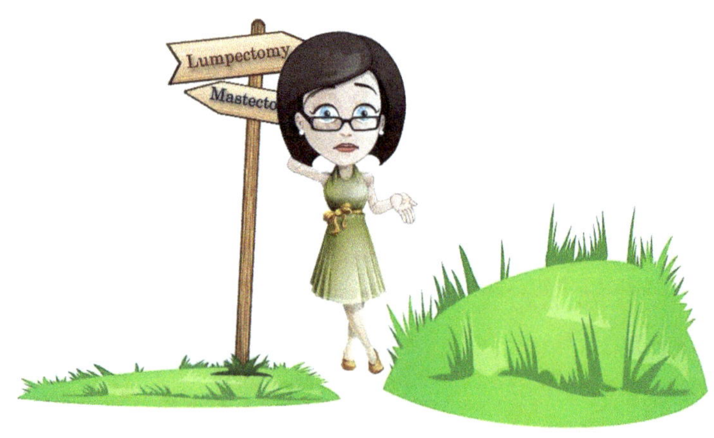

You will usually find yourself in one of these three categories. Which one are you?

- "I want this thing (my breast) gone!" It's a traitorous troublemaker. I'm done with it. I am done breastfeeding. No one is looking at the darn thing anymore (or the person that does, loves me with or without my breasts).

- "Um . . . um . . . what should I do, doc? This one is a doozy." Well, as long as you don't *need* a mastectomy, I recommend lumpectomy. Lumpectomy means less surgery (less risk), offers an easier recovery, and results in less body-image issues. Of course, lumpectomy isn't perfect either. Let's face it, this whole process, at times, is going to seem like a crapshoot.

- "You can't take my breast! Doc, I need my breasts, and that's that!"

You can go online and find a million pictures of mastectomies, reconstructed breasts, lumpectomies, etc. Just remember everyone scars differently. Everyone's body is different. It's not like ordering off a menu. It's more like ordering a dress online. Results will vary!

One more important word: recurrence. Specifically, local recurrence (meaning in the breast after lumpectomy or on the chest wall or skin after mastectomy). What's the rate, doc? Well, that is not an easy answer. Because it's different depending on who you are, your age, your type of cancer, if your cancer has spread to your lymph nodes, and so on. You get the point. We can look at studies of large groups of women with different types of cancer and come up with numbers, but do those accurately depict you and your risk after a lumpectomy or mastectomy? Nope. Generally, lumpectomy with radiation is thought to have a higher recurrence rate by some amount (because, let's face it, there's a whole lot more breast left behind after lumpectomy).

Does the thought of a breast cancer recurrence have you breathing into a paper bag? You might just be a champion worrier who will dwell in the small percentage difference. I know who you are! There is no judgment here. I have been known to be an imaginative worrier myself! If you know that you will be entirely undone by the thought of not doing everything you possibly can to prevent a future breast cancer, then you may consider mastectomy. Is anything here straightforward? Ahh!

Mastectomy: What to Expect

1. You will need four weeks of recovery time (six weeks with reconstruction).

2. You may go home the same day or stay one night in the hospital. If you have reconstruction, you may stay for several days, depending on the type of reconstruction.

3. You will have a drain for one to four weeks (or maybe more). This stinker is a pain in the butt. But believe me, it's your friend. It doesn't come out until the output is low. For some, that happens at one week. For others, it may take more than four weeks.

4. You will likely be numb on your chest wall—forever.

5. You can get immediate reconstruction (performed at the time of mastectomy) or delayed reconstruction (which can happen in months or even years after your surgery).

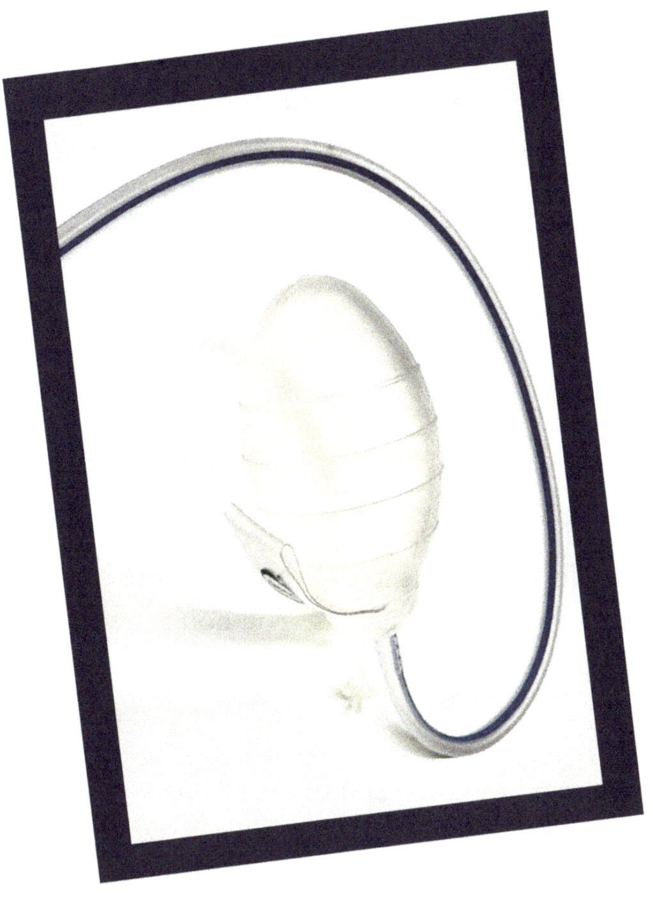

Oh, and that pesky armpit fat? Girlfriend, that's not breast, and it's still going to be there. Remember that time the guy in your office shaved his head, and you noticed all those upper neck rolls for the first time . . . well, that could happen to you. You may notice some fluff that your breasts were camouflaging for you. And you may notice your upper abdomen in a way that you have not experienced since before puberty. Let's face it; it was probably cuter then, but times have changed. Also, you are not to be defined by your physical body, so practice a bit of self-love and self-acceptance. This kindness toward yourself will aid your healing in many ways: physical, mental, emotional.

"Okay, so whatever. I pad my bra."

Prosthetics

Post-surgery, your old bra will probably not cut it anymore. But don't sweat it! There are many fantastic breast prostheses, bras with built-in breasts, and other options. You may have to travel to the nearest city, but there are breast/bra mavericks that can be the Q to your James Bond! (All right, your fancy bra isn't going to double as a Wi-Fi hotspot, but you will look damn good in clothes.) To give you some in-depth information here, I have enlisted my own Q! Jump to the Expert Extras chapter at the end of the book when you are ready for "Bras and Prosthetics and Posture, Oh My" by Victoria Hand on page 188.

When all is said and done, preparing yourself for a mastectomy is something akin to preparing someone for childbirth. We all experience life differently. It can be painful (although for some, the psychological pain may be the hardest to deal with). Frankly, though, it is not something you can prepare someone for; it must be lived.

Prophylactic Mastectomy

"What about the other one, Doc?"

There is no survival benefit to removing a healthy breast in a lady without a pathogenic/deleterious genetic variant. No survival benefit. With few exceptions, the recommendation from a cancer perspective is: You don't need to get rid of your breast . . . period. Keep that tata. Own it. Get it a yearly mammogram, and enjoy it!

However, some women feel that symmetry is essential and opt for a bilateral mastectomy with reconstruction so that they "match." Some women have had it "up to here" with this whole nonsense, and they want to take their risk of breast cancer as close to zero as possible. Some women have just made up their minds that they are going flat . . . period, no discussion. Some women are fed up with annual screening and want to be done with all that imaging business. Everyone has a different reason for bilateral mastectomy. Most surgeons will oblige you and remove your non-cancer breast when your cancer-containing breast is removed. But you should know a few things. First, the risk of breast cancer after a mastectomy is not zero. Second, insurance may not pay for the removal of a healthy breast. And finally, again, there is no survival benefit (i.e. you won't live longer).

Woah, doc, run me back through that first one? Number one, the risk of breast cancer after a mastectomy is not 0 percent. There is no 100 percent guarantee you won't get breast cancer again. Sorry for the bad news! The risk is in the 1 to 5 percent range, depending on where you look. Now, if you are scratching your head thinking, Why is it not zero? The answer is simple. The breast tissue doesn't sit in the skin like a ping-pong ball in a sock. No, breasts must be complicated little (or big) troublemakers. They are more like pie filling in a pie crust. You cannot separate the two completely. They are mushed together, and your surgeon is not going to leave you with an open wound where your breast was. We need to leave skin to close you up, and that skin will have some pie filling (breast cells) stuck to the crust (skin). And those cells, although small in volume, will carry a lifelong risk of making trouble!

Studies have shown that women way overestimate their risk of getting breast cancer again. If you leave your healthy breast in place, there is a less than 1 percent chance per year of developing cancer (maybe even considerably less). Period. Most of the time, that tata will be the good one, and you will have had only one naughty troublemaker breast. If you have been paying attention, you may have noticed that the odds of dying from breast cancer are small if you are undergoing regular screening imaging. Ipso-facto, if you leave the healthy breast in place, yes, it may get cancer (rarely). But, if you continue yearly (or more frequent, if your doctor requests it) screening, the odds are that the cancer will be found when it is curable (but yes . . . you would be back on the cancer treatment train again).

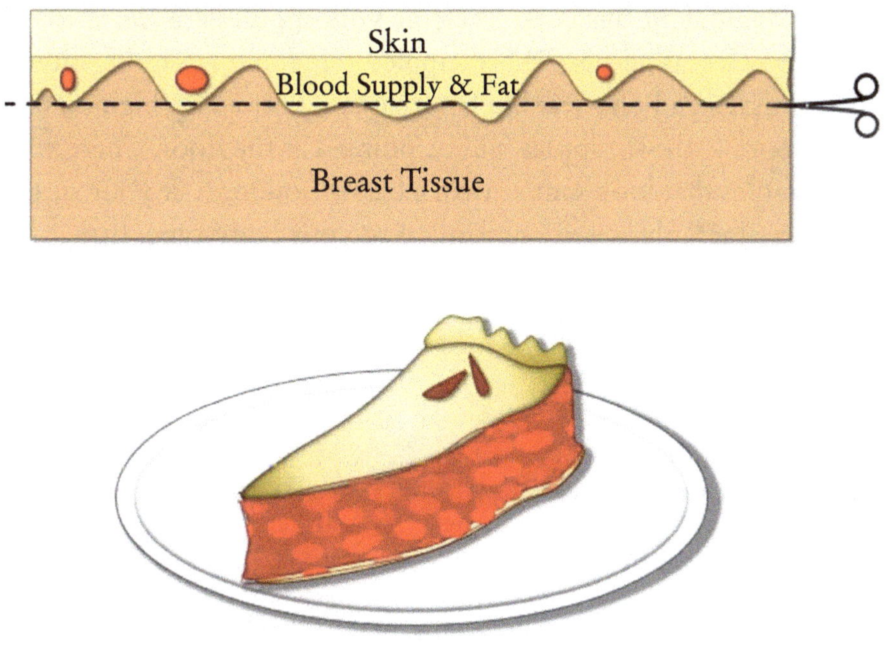

Now, let's look at pathogenic genetic variant carriers. There is a sizeable body of research here. Some studies focused on women who had their breasts removed before a cancer diagnosis (prophylactically). Some focused on women with cancer who underwent a bilateral mastectomy. By and large, bilateral mastectomy decreased these ladies' risk of cancer by 90 to 95 percent. Bilateral mastectomy is generally believed to translate into a survival advantage for BRCA1 pathogenic genetic variant carriers (maybe less so for BRCA2 mutation carriers). Also of note, if you are a pathogenic variant carrier, removal of the ovaries has a survival advantage from both an ovarian and breast cancer perspective. However, the breast cancer benefit is limited to those women who undergo removal of the ovaries during the premenopausal years, usually around age forty, go figure.

If you have decided mastectomy is for you, you may be wondering, Can I keep my nipples?

The short answer is: maybe. First, your cancer cannot be snuggled up next to or near the nipple. Remember, we need to get the whole cancer out! Second, we must ask, "Can a plastic surgeon give me a good cosmetic result?" In general, nipple-sparing mastectomy is reserved for smaller-chested women. Let's take an extreme example to highlight this issue. Imagine your nipples are closer to your navel than your clavicles. Where are those nipples going to be pointing after you remove the breast tissue and place an implant that is anchored up high on the chest wall? The floor . . . those nipples will be pointed at the floor. There will be excess skin and nipples that look sadder than a basset hound. Ask your surgeon and plastic surgeon what might work according to your body type. But understand that there are limits. If you just love your nipples (we all have our things), then there may be options like free nipple transfer (talk with the plastic surgeon).

"All right! Green light for a lumpectomy. Now it's full steam ahead, doc! When's the big day?"

Whoa, cowgirl. Unless your mass is something that you can easily feel, you might be skipping a step. How is your surgeon going to find the needle in that haystack of yours? You may be thinking, "No worries, doc, they placed a clip at the time of biopsy." Unfortunately, that clip is the needle in the haystack, so we are back where we started. Most clips placed at the time of a biopsy are teeny-tiny, itty-bitty little pieces of metal that are great if you are looking at a mammogram, but not so great when looking at a person. Have no fear. We will find it! But you will need some way for the surgeon to *localize* or find your cancer.

There are a ton of ways to do this. But the gist is, something else is going into your breast that serves as a map or homing beacon for the surgeon. There are two main ways this is done. Either an additional clip is placed in the breast, or a wire is placed.

Fancy clips usually make noise when the surgeon waves their magic science wand (think of a metal detector on the beach that beeps louder the closer the wand gets to the clip). If you don't get a fancy clip, you get a wire. A literal piece of metal wire is placed in the breast like a spear right through the center of the cancer. The surgeon follows that wire and removes that cancer like a lollipop on a stick. If you are thinking, "This is bogus! Why didn't some fancy clip get placed in the first place? And no, I do not want a wire sticking out of my breast!" Well, there are a ton of biopsies performed that turn out to be nothing. And those women don't need thousands of dollars in fancy, expensive clips hanging out in their breast. And think, if they do one day need a lumpectomy, they don't want a whole bunch of false

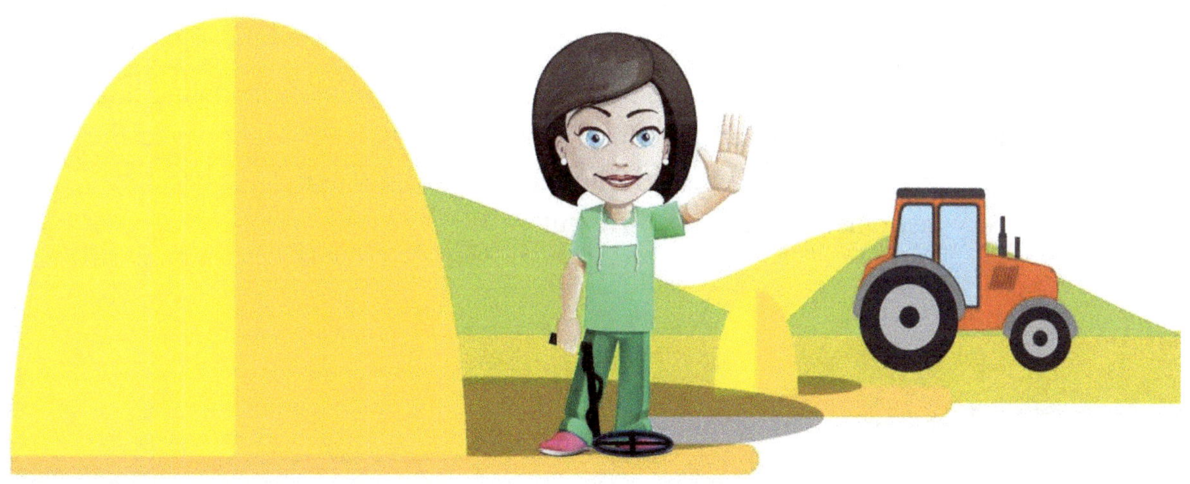

alarms from old clips beeping all over the place. Also, all those fancy clips aren't needed for mastectomy. So why put in a fancy clip that will never be used?

That being said, sometimes, at the discretion of the radiologist, a fancy clip may be placed upfront. And if that is you, disregard the previous paragraph.

If you are having one of the many types of special clips placed in your breast, this usually occurs days to weeks before the procedure (and the flavors are: radioactive, magnetic, radar, or RFID). If you have a wire placed, that is done on the day of surgery. (No, you won't have to walk around with some strange breast piercing hanging out of you for days on end.) Whatever the technique, the results are the same. Your surgeon can find the cancer and get it out!

Oncoplastic Lumpectomy

Depending on how good you are at looking at the glass as "half full," this cancer business may not be all bad. (All right, this is a stretch, but stay with me.) That creepy cancer may actually be the impetus for a top-shelf renovation! Breast lift or breast reduction, here we come! Depending on some factors (best left to an in-depth discussion with your breast surgeon and plastic surgeon), you may be a candidate for a breast lift or breast reduction at the time of your cancer surgery. And we are talking about both sides, not just the cancer side. Silver-lining alert! If you are one of those ladies that always wanted some remodeling but didn't want to shell out the bucks, your cancer may have just paved the way for a freebie. (Check with the doctor's office about costs because every insurance company is different.)

Lumpectomy: What to Expect

1. You will need two weeks of recovery time.

2. You will go home the same day.

3. You may have scar tissue that you can feel like a mass.

4. You may feel or hear some "sloshing" of fluid. (In the same way that a blister accumulates fluid, so, too, will the empty space where your cancer was. As a result, you will have a fluid collection. The fancy medical term for this is seroma.) This can, in some cases, be persistent.

5. There is the possibility of "positive margins," which would necessitate a return to the OR (see: "What the Heck is a Margin? on page 63"). Woah! Full stop here. You're telling me I may have to go back to the OR? Yes I am. And it can happen for several reasons in ladies undergoing both lumpectomy or mastectomy (see insert "Going back to the OR" on page 62).

6. You may have tenderness or some pain that persists.

"Oncoplastic Reconstruction after Lumpectomy"

by Maryann Martinovic, MD

Too big? Too loose? Too sad? Oncoplastic reconstruction may be Goldilocks' answer to your breast woes!

If you are a candidate for a lumpectomy, a plastic surgeon may be able to put Humpty Dumpty back together again in a new-and-improved way. Oncoplastic reconstruction is a fancy term for stealing or borrowing tissue from another part of the breast to fill in the hole created by the lumpectomy. This may require removing extra skin or breast tissue. Or it may just mean rearranging what breast tissue you have left and placing it into a better position. In doing such, we may be able to make a G-cup breast into a cute C cup. If sagging is more of an issue than size, nipples that once grazed your belly may now be restored to a youthful pre-pregnancy, pre-aging state. Often, women have considered improving their breast shape or size prior to a cancer diagnosis but never moved forward with it. Now they may get a chance to get some perks (pun intended) out of this whole process!

While this may sound so very tempting, it is not always sunshine and roses. Women who have lumpectomies generally require radiation treatment to the affected breast after their surgery. And radiation can sometimes change the appearance of all that hard work the plastic surgeon has done to give you a new and improved breast. But rest assured, plastic surgeons have lots of tricks up their sleeves. Other procedures can often be done later down the line to make improvements and alterations. One commonly offered alteration is fat grafting; this is where unwanted fat gets taken from your belly pooch and repurposed in your breast. It's a win-win. And best of all, your insurance generally covers these procedures.

If your breast surgeon thinks that you are a good match for a lumpectomy, be sure to consult with a plastic surgeon to discuss oncoplastic reconstruction. At the end of the day, you may walk away with the breasts of your dreams!

Going back to the OR

Round Two!

"Doc, I never wanted to go to the OR in the first place, and I sure don't want to go back again!" Well, there are several reasons you may end up back in the OR.

1. Your lymph nodes are positive (there is cancer in them), and now your surgeon says you need an axillary dissection. While positive lymph nodes certainly don't always require a return trip back to the OR, it may be in the cards for you, depending on some very specific scenarios. See the lymph node section starting on page 67 for some more details.

2. Your "margin" is positive, and now you need to go back to remove more tissue to make sure no cancer is left in the breast. See the next section for more information.

3. A complication. The most common complication that leads back to the OR is significant bleeding (you go back to the OR ASAP). Also, very rarely you may have to go back to the OR for infection, wound breakdown, or skin necrosis. (Yep, it's as bad as it sounds: dead skin resulting from inadequate blood supply.)

What the Heck Is a "Margin?"

Getting All the Cancer Out!

Unfortunately, cancer is not a perfectly round ball. It usually grows in some amorphous stellate shape (think star blob). And although many surgeons aim to remove a buffer of healthy tissue around the cancer, there is no guarantee on the day of surgery that the crab cancer is going to be removed in its entirety. (I know, you're thinking, "What the ever-loving, bummer news are you giving me now?") Sometimes after lumpectomy, there is what is called a "positive margin," which means that there is cancer at the cut edge. This means that there could be cancer left in your body. Now, before you fire your surgeon, there are some things to know! The positive margin rate is somewhere in the 15 to 20 percent range nationally. And yes, the scientists are on it. (trying to bring this to zero, but we just aren't there yet!) So, let's talk "margins." There is a balance to maintain. The goal is to remove the cancer without removing too much breast. Enter the Goldilocks story of the breast.

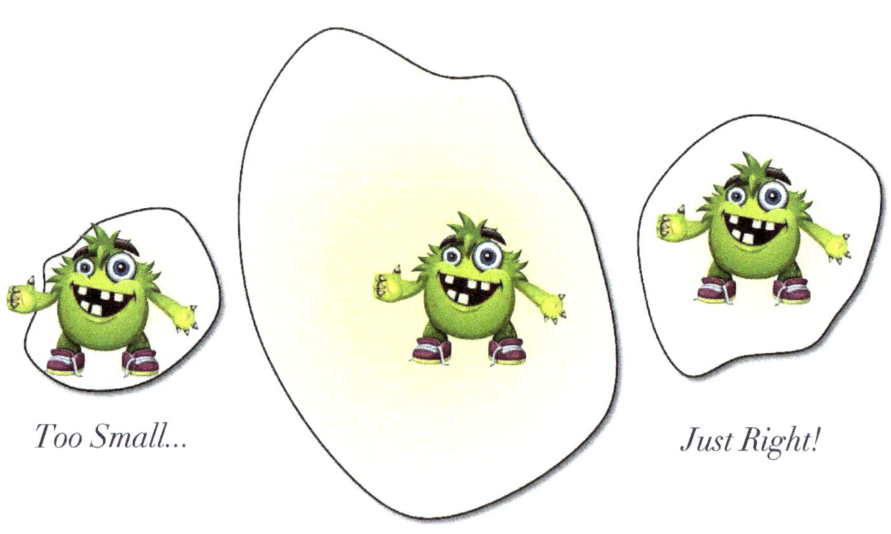

Bring in the Plastic Surgeon!

A Quick Overview of Reconstruction Options

Now we have gone and done it. We've opened another Pandora's Box: reconstruction. It's simple to say, "Make me some breasts, doc!" But it's another thing to navigate through this next jungle of decisions! And remember, reconstruction is considered "elective" or optional when it comes to your physical health and cancer survival. This means that the risks and benefits profile is slightly different (see the risks and benefits section on page 48).

I am not discounting the importance of psychological health and the clear benefits of reconstruction—not by any means—but it's not considered *lifesaving*. Therefore, it's considered "elective." Because of this, you need to meet some basic health parameters to qualify. These parameters can vary by surgeon, but many plastic surgeons have some hard rules to limit putting you at too much risk. Let's face it: this is going to be a partnership. Although you may be shoveling coal in the fire and going full steam ahead with high potential risk, your partner (the plastic surgeon) needs to be on board with you. If this sounds unfair, then imagine hearing about a plastic surgeon killing people with facelifts. Does that sound like a good plastic surgeon? Nope. Okay, then realize that a plastic surgeon doesn't want these outcomes for you and needs to make sure that you will heal well and survive the surgery. They want to set you up for success. After all, you have this whole other thing to focus on, like completing your breast cancer treatment. You don't want to end up in some nightmare situation (wounds, bleeding, or worse). Not only does that sound bad, but it also delays important things like—I don't know—chemotherapy.

Now some hard stops may be things like being overweight or a smoker. If you're currently smoking while reading this or have been trying to lose weight for years and now you are spiraling into a dark place—stop! These dedicated doctors aren't trying to dash your dreams! But remember that neither you nor your plastic surgeon wants your reconstruction to fail, right? Part of their job is knowing when to say "no" or "not right now."

Reconstruction can be done at any time after surgery. Take a deep breath, now take another. If you are smoking and you are ready to quit, do it now. Here is that extra motivation that you needed. You may be realizing that you will need a plastic surgeon that you like (and if you love them, that's even better). Reconstruction can be immediate (at the time of mastectomy) or delayed (at some time after your mastectomy).

The two main types of reconstruction are, at the most basic level: implant-based or tissue-based. (In rearranging bits of you, it may sound like arts and crafts in a horror flick. But you may just get a tummy tuck with your new tatas!)

Implant-based:

First, there's no good evidence to say that implants make you sick (clearly, there are women out there who disagree). Second, there's a ton of buzz about implants causing a particular type of breast cancer. Yes, it's true. But gee whiz, is it rare! You are more likely to be struck by lightning, which, interestingly, is 1 in 12,000 per year on a quick Google search. (Disclaimer: I am no lightning expert. The incidence of this particular breast cancer, related to implants, is less than one per million in some reports to 1 in 30,000 in other reports.) When we compare implant-based reconstruction to the other option (using your own

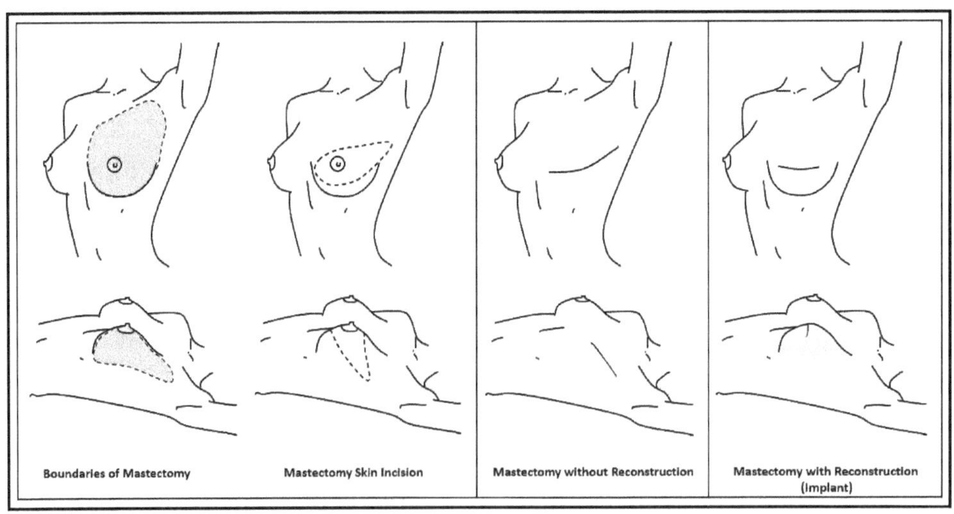

tissue), the hospital stay is shorter and the complication rate is lower. But there are certainly some trade-offs. Most women don't get implants the same day as their mastectomy. They get tissue expanders (which are, for all intents and purposes, deflated implants). These slowly get expanded over time (think multiple visits to your favorite plastic surgeon). They eventually get swapped out for an implant. Now if all this seems like a lot of extra steps, let me explain why.

First, what happens when you squeeze your thumbnail? It turns white. This is because the pressure of the squeeze forces all the blood out. (Just do it to illustrate the point. C'mon, let's get interactive.) Well, all that skin on your chest just lost its deep blood supply (any blood supply coming from the underlying breast). For the gardeners out there, we just disrupted the deep root system (note, this is not the last gardening analogy). If you push on this skin with the pressure of an implant (just like when you pushed on your thumb) that skin is going to turn white, and the blood supply is going to be even more tenuous. And skin (or really any body part) without a blood supply dies. Yes, that is as bad as it sounds! So there is a good reason for the whole rigmarole. That being said, some women may be candidates for "direct to implant" reconstruction. (The risks and benefits of this are something that are decided on a case-by-case basis. If your plastic surgeon pushes back, think "dead skin" and consider their expert opinion!)

Tissue-based:

This is also not a straightforward reconstruction. I think you are starting to see a trend here. I get it, and that is why you need your A-team! So, if you aren't interested in implants, there are some minimum requirements for tissue-based reconstruction. First, you need to have enough (but not too much) tissue to move and create a breast. I know, those picky Goldilocks plastic surgeons. And you need to be able to tolerate an extensive surgery. We are sometimes talking all-day surgery (and not an eight-hour workday either), with up to four days in the hospital and some serious potential complications. You've got your TRAM flaps (free and pedicle), DIEP flaps, and a whole host of other possible flaps. If your head is spinning and you're totally overwhelmed, that's okay! Talk to your surgeon. They will let you know what you are or aren't a good candidate for!

Finally, we can combine flaps and implants. Some women may be in need of some extra skin or some extra fullness for all sorts of reasons. Enter the latissimus flap with an implant. It is just as it sounds. We are bringing skin and muscle from the back so that you have an envelope to place the implant in and then bringing in the implant so that there is something in that envelope. Overall, there are certainly women with all sorts of combinations of flaps and implants out there.

I hate to break it to you, but life is not perfect, as you may have already guessed. Sometimes things don't go as planned. (Do they ever?) You may wake up without your planned reconstruction. Pick your chin up off the floor. This is rare, but it happens. There are many reasons for this. If you were planning on getting implant-based reconstruction and the plastic surgeon is worried about the blood supply to the skin, they may want to place that expander in a couple of weeks after the skin has had a chance to get used to its new situation (remember, no one wants dead skin). Or maybe things did not go as expected with your cancer operation. Some plastic surgeons won't place expanders if the lymph nodes are unexpectedly positive and radiation is expected. Why? Because radiation and expanders (depending on timing) can be like oil and water; they just don't mix well. Like everything here, there are infinite details and caveats to rules that go into making these decisions, and there's no way to cover them all. But you get the gist. Things change, they don't always go as planned, but your surgeons are always trying to make the best decisions with the information that they have!

Lymph Nodes

I'm Ticklish! Stay Out of My Armpits!

So cancer can be a wily beast, and if it's going to try to hitchhike its way out of the breast, there are two main ways to do it—the blood vessels or the lymphatic channels. The *what* channels, you ask?

Time for a crash course in some science stuff.

What the heck are lymph nodes?

First, let's start with blood vessels. Their job is to carry blood, which contains oxygen, nutrients, and fluid. Now remember that people need to drink fluids to stay hydrated. (Dehydration makes us feel crummy and can eventually cause death! But why?) All our cells need water. Vessels serve to drop off the water with all that other stuff. But what happens to all that fluid? Well, it goes into cells that need it (they drink it up . . . ahh!), but there's extra water, and it needs to be recycled back into the blood vessels. Ta-da! That's what the lymph system is for. It scrounges up all that fluid and runs it through some fancy little water filters (lymph nodes) before the fluid gets dumped back into the blood vessels. Therefore, if we lose our lymph system, we become puffy like the Michelin Man!

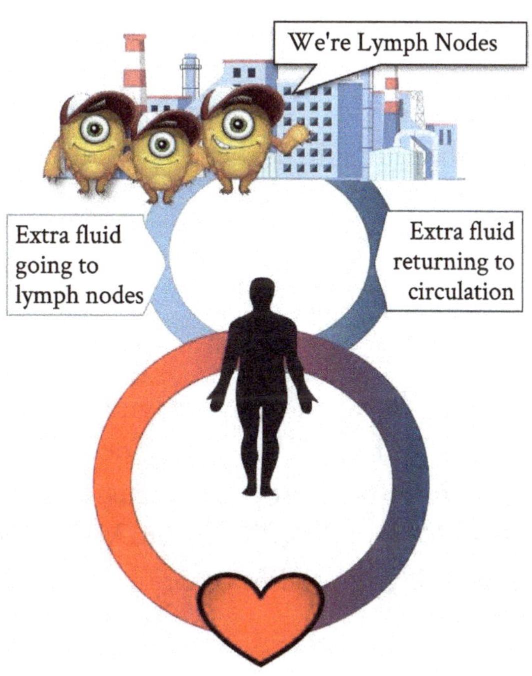

These lymph node water filters are a little more complex than your standard charcoal filter. They are also packed with key immune system components. They surveil the fluid for invaders or cancers and attack and destroy (which makes sense if you have ever notice swollen lymph nodes when you have been sick in the past).

If the cancer beasties in your breast try to hitchhike out on the lymph highways (or water recycling pipes in your breast), they will likely get caught in the first lymph node (water filter) that they see. There is a caveat though. Anyone with a water filter knows that these things are not 100 percent efficacious, and the same goes for your body. We also know that if it does leave on these lymphatic highways, these highways are most commonly headed straight for the armpit area. That's why we check these armpit lymph nodes for cancer at the same time that we are removing the cancer from your breast. We need to know if this is a traveling cancer or a sedentary cancer because the answer will change treatment recommendations.

Do you have cancer in your lymph nodes?

STOP! Answer this question before you read on and become completely confused! There's enough reading to do here without muddying the waters with someone else's problems.

If your answer is, "No, I do not have cancer in my lymph nodes," then read this section.

If your answer is "Yes, I do have cancer in my lymph nodes," then you will likely skip this section and go to "axillary lymph node dissection" on page 74. However, individualized treatment plans discussed with your doctor could still include the information in this section. My recommendation is to wait for this discussion with your doctor before you go delving into extra information!

If your answer is "Maybe," then it's because the radiologists are worried your lymph nodes look suspicious, but a biopsy of your lymph node was negative for cancer. You may be thinking, I am in the clear, right? Not so fast, speed demon. Slow down and read the section on sampling error on page 40 and circle back around. Got it? You see, a negative biopsy doesn't rule out cancer. You will still need a sentinel lymph node biopsy.

DCIS: Stage 0 Disease

Yes, you have breast cancer, but it's not the kind of breast cancer that hitchhikes its way out of the breast. It's a homebody, as far as we know from the biopsy. But remember that this biopsy was just a sample (see sampling error section again on page 40 if you need a brushup). We treat this cancer just the same as an invasive cancer, with one caveat: Most surgeons don't sample the lymph nodes if you are getting a lumpectomy. But, due to sampling error, we will still need to sample nodes if you are getting a mastectomy. Why? If your lumpectomy pathology ends up "upstaging" you to an invasive cancer, the breast, with all its lymphatic highways, is still in place, and a sentinel lymph node biopsy can be performed as a second surgery. If, however, you are getting a mastectomy for your DCIS and invasive cancer is found after the surgery is done, it's really hard to go back for a sentinel lymph node biopsy. Why? You just demolished all of the highways. So, rather than being stuck in this situation, you will usually get a sentinel lymph node biopsy if you are getting a mastectomy for DCIS.

Sentinel Lymph Node Biopsy

"Is there cancer in my lymph nodes?"

What is a sentinel lymph node biopsy? You know I like analogies, and the way I think about this one is as follows:

Your breast is like an island, and your lymph nodes in your armpit are also like an island. Got it? Start drawing in the lymph highways on the islands, then draw a couple of bridges between the two. Put some gatekeeper nodes at the bridges on the lymph node side. Let's call them "sentry" or sentinel lymph nodes. These little buddies will protect the lymph node island from cancer and catch and detain any cancer cells headed their way. At this point, we are going to have to dabble in some very brief historical context. We have known for a long time that breast cancer goes to lymph nodes under the armpit. (For you curious cats, head to the "Sassy Story: They Did What?" section at the end of this chapter.) And for a long time, we were concerned about this and "bombed the whole lymph node island into oblivion." Thankfully, though, some brilliant people in the 1990s decided that there had to be a better way. Enter the "sentinel lymph node biopsy." Remember those sentry (or gatekeeper) nodes? Some smart people figured out how to find and remove just those guys and leave the island intact!

How on earth do we find these magical gatekeepers? Well, we use the lymph system itself. On the day of surgery, you will get injections in your breast. (Many surgeons use a radioactive material and a blue dye, but there are certainly other types of tracers.) These tracers are taken up by the lymph highways in the breast, they cross those bridges, and then they get stuck in those little gatekeeper nodes. This allows the surgeon to find those little suckers using a Geiger counter (think something akin to a metal detector on the beach), and they also use their eyes to look for blue. Anything that is "hot" with radioactive material and/or blue with dye is removed. The surgeon then takes a feel of the area, and anything suspicious also gets removed. These nodes are all sent to the pathologist to answer the question: Is there cancer in the lymph nodes?

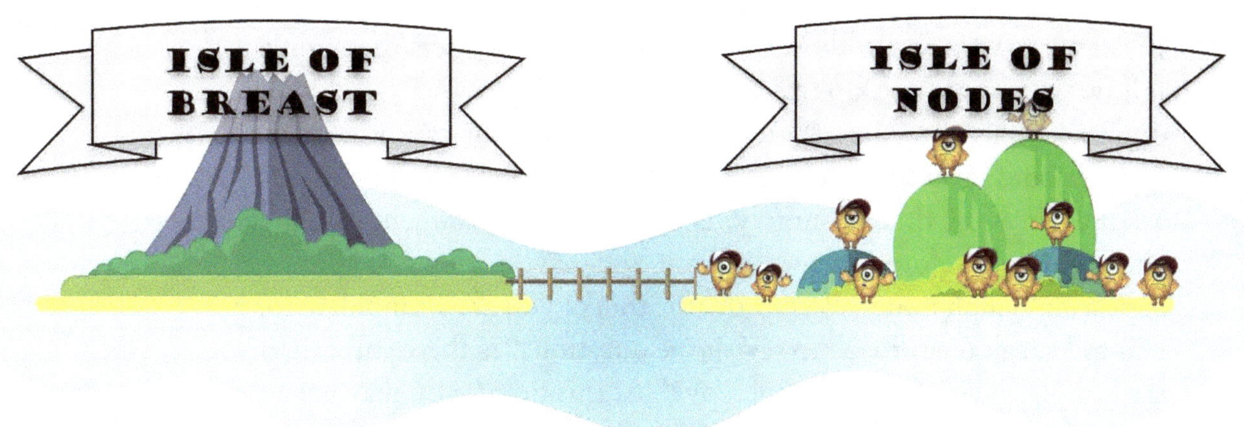

Cancer Beasties on the Move

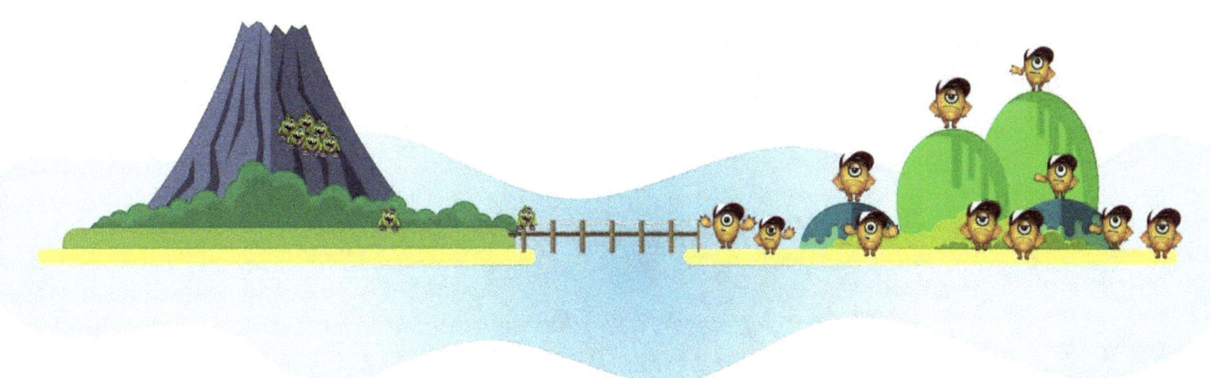

Sentinel Lymph Node Biopsy

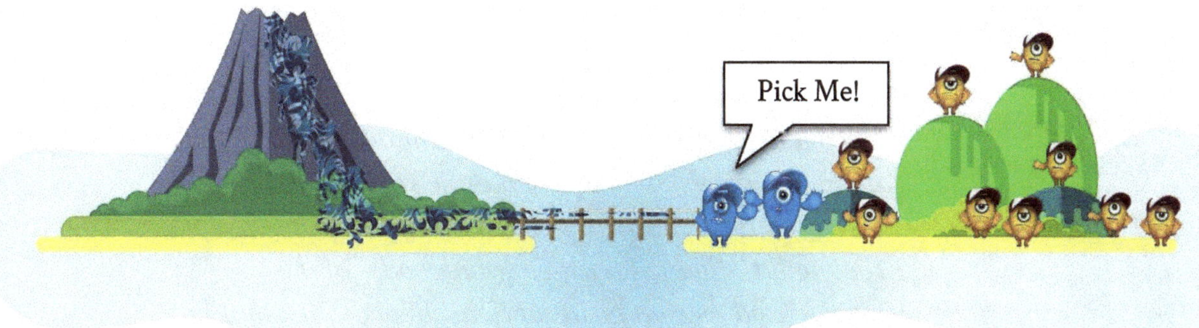

In case you were one of those node-positive rule breakers that didn't follow the prompt to skip this section, you now know why you likely don't need this procedure. You already know that the cancer is in your lymph nodes. You have the answer to this question, so there's no need to ask it again at the time of surgery. Unless . . . your treatment plan includes chemotherapy before surgery, and you only have a couple of abnormal appearing lymph nodes. If your doctor thinks you are a candidate for a tailored surgical approach to revisit the question, "Is there still cancer in the lymph nodes after chemotherapy?" At this point, you may get a sentinel node biopsy; this is getting into the science-based decisions that are best left to a discussion with your surgeon.

Now, suppose your sentinel lymph nodes are negative. In that case, we will go ahead and believe that your cancer is a sedentary little crab with no aspirations of traveling abroad. Let's call this a wrap, tie up some loose ends, and proceed. You can skip the section on axillary lymph node dissection.

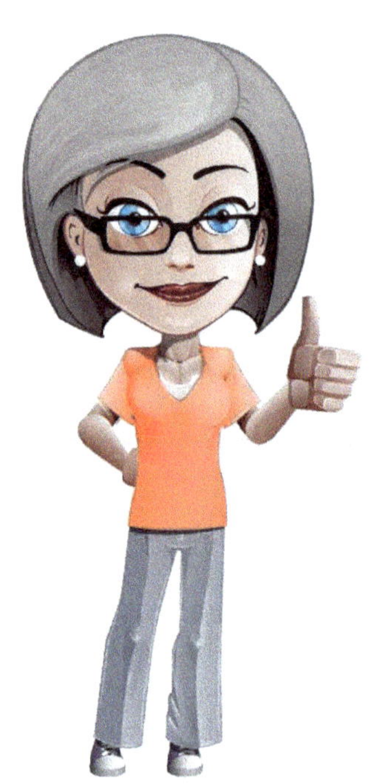

Guidelines for Choosing Wisely®

There are times in life when getting older isn't so glamorous. And then there are small, shining moments when being a little more mature gives you an upper hand. Here is one such instance. First, you need to be seventy or older. Second, you need a small, well-behaved invasive cancer (hormone-positive, HER2 negative). Third, you need normal lymph nodes on exam or imaging. If you check all of these boxes, your surgeon may discuss leaving that whole lymph node sampling business out! No, we are certainly not putting you out to pasture, and age is just a number. But studies in women who meet all these criteria found no increased risk of local-regional recurrence (cancer coming back in the breast or lymph nodes of the armpit) and no change in survival! Boom! Stick that in your seventy-plus-year hat and march on!

Axillary Lymph Node Dissection

Take 'Em All!

So your answer is, "Yes, I have cancer in my lymph nodes." Maybe you like to travel, or at least you always wanted to . . . Why does this cancer have to have that in common with you?

If you have cancer in your lymph nodes, your surgeon is going to talk to you about axillary lymph node dissection. These nodes can be found before surgery, at the time of surgery during sentinel lymph node biopsy, or after surgery when the pathologists review all the slides.

With every rule, there are exceptions, and these exceptions change and flex with new information. Here is where the details get tricky, though, and you need a specialist to navigate these waters. Some exceptions right now:

- This "rule" trumps all other rules, and there are not many exceptions. If you had chemotherapy before surgery, you will need an axillary dissection if even a single cancer cell is found in your lymph nodes. Why? Because this cancer was resistant to chemotherapy. If a woman has even one cancer cell remaining in her sentinel nodes after chemotherapy, there is a high chance of cancer in additional nodes (60 percent in some studies). The whole island has to go.

- Lumpectomy ladies who didn't get chemotherapy before surgery get a free pass on one or two positive nodes (with some exceptions)—no more surgery for you, chicka.

- Everyone who didn't get chemotherapy before surgery gets a free pass on micromets—aka micrometastasis (these are teeny-tiny little bits of cancer in the nodes).

- Everyone who didn't get chemotherapy before surgery gets a free pass on what we call "isolated tumor cells." I know it sounds crazy, but we try to pretend that they aren't there at all. You are technically considered "node-negative." (Those little cancer cells don't even count!) Before you throw in the towel on this "medicine stuff" that no longer makes sense, let me try to explain. These cells are only able to be found nowadays using special stains. These cells were not consistently detected prior to this stain. And, a plethora of breast cancer studies were done before these stains came along! So we asked, "Do these cells matter?" We concluded that these isolated cells have no clinical significance. This is doctor-speak for, "They don't have any impact on you, your future, your recurrence rate, or your treatment recommendations."

And, of course, as the medical community continues to improve treatment strategies, management will change—for the better! Thank goodness for science and clinical trials and the ladies willing to pay it forward!

"What Does Axillary Lymph Node Dissection Actually Mean?"

Ladies, I know what you might be thinking. Lymph nodes are like a bunch of grapes, right? You just pluck them out and count them as you go. Nope, the body just isn't like that! The best way to understand the mess of lymph nodes under your armpit is to imagine a bowl of tapioca pudding (if you haven't experienced this yet, give it a try!). The surgeon's job is to scrape the bowl or container of tapioca pudding clean. That guy or gal has no idea how many tapioca balls are in that pudding. It would be like guessing how many jelly beans are in the jar. Who knows? All the surgeon knows on the day of surgery is that they must scrape the bowl clean.

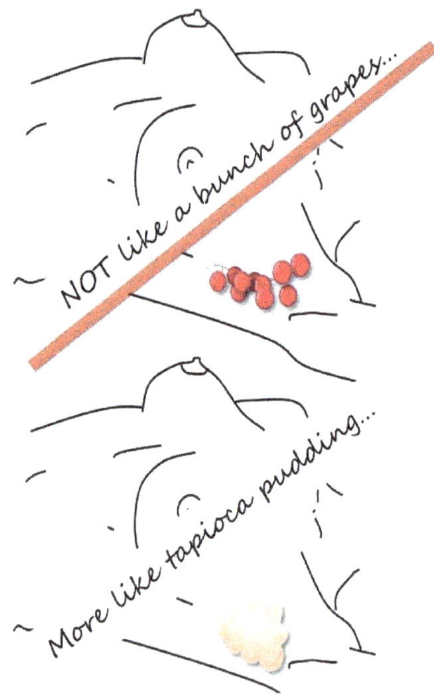

The pathology lab's job is to sift through all the pudding (fat) and pick out the tapioca balls (lymph nodes). They count them, process them, and take a close look at them under the microscope. They then take a tally of how many nodes were removed and how many are positive.

Some of you may wonder, Why don't you just take out all the lymph nodes each time? What's the big deal? One word: lymphedema (arm swelling). "Shut the front door!" You've got cancer traveling from base camp in the breast to the lymph nodes. Now, someone has the gall to tell you that removing these nodes to remove the cancer means that you also have a chance of permanent, non-curable arm swelling? "Any more good news for me today, doc?" An axillary lymph node dissection has a 30 percent chance of lymphedema, called arm swelling. This rate increases with radiation and other risk factors. But fear not, although this is not a curable condition, there are certainly treatment options. Think of it like diabetes; management is key! Also, like all things in life, lymphedema is a spectrum of disease. There are some women with only a slight difference in arm size (mild disease), and there are also women with a defunctionalized arm (the most severe form of lymphedema, and luckily this is the minority of women).

Lymphedema

This section is not just for the ladies who win the axillary lymph node dissection lottery. The other risks are mastectomy, obesity, and radiation. The rate of lymphedema after a sentinel lymph node biopsy is up to 5 percent. So this is a must-read section for just about everyone.

Lymphedema is a spectrum. Some have it bad, some not so much. But in the end, remember this: early intervention is key! There are occupational and physical therapists that specialize in lymphedema resulting from breast cancer treatment. If you are lucky enough to have one in your locale, find them!

Most cases (80 percent or more) will start within three years of surgery. But that means that up to 20 percent of women will have symptoms that don't start for more than three years.

Just in case you were skimming and your mind was wandering, remember:

Early intervention is key

Early intervention is key.

Early intervention is key.

So, here's the lowdown. This is still a developing area of medicine. The definition of lymphedema is not quite nailed down. Do we define it by it's symptoms? Do we define it as an absolute size increase of the arm? Well, we aren't sure yet. But many people talk about it in terms of stages. There are stages of lymphedema. Yes . . . stages again.

Stage 0: "Something just ain't right, but my arm looks just fine." Ladies at this stage of lymphedema feel changes in their arm. Some experience this as a tired or heavy arm or an odd sensation like numbness and tingling. But their arm looks normal. You can be stalled at this stage for months or years. Physical therapy is going to help you stay in this stage.

Stage 1: "There is some swelling, but it comes and goes." At this stage, your arm looks different . . . sometimes. If you leave your arm elevated like you desperately want the teacher to call on you—for a long time—your swelling will disappear. This is treatable; no permanent damage is done. Get on it, girl, and see your local PT.

Stage 2: "This swelling does not ever go away, and something weird is happening to my skin." Damage done to the skin at this stage can't be undone. But before it gets any worse, seek help, seek help, and seek help!

Stage 3: This stage is rare. It conjures up the statement: "Well, this just isn't my arm anymore. It's something else." Although this is rare, some women will end up with a very large, very altered arm.

Once you start down the path of these stages, your goal is to stop at the lowest possible stage. The only way to do this is to invest the time in your self-care and get help (I know . . . broken record).

If you are heading for an axillary lymph node dissection, skip to the "expert opinion" chapter and read "Lymphedema" by Dr. Lisa Spiguel on page 184.

Thoughts and Questions About Surgery

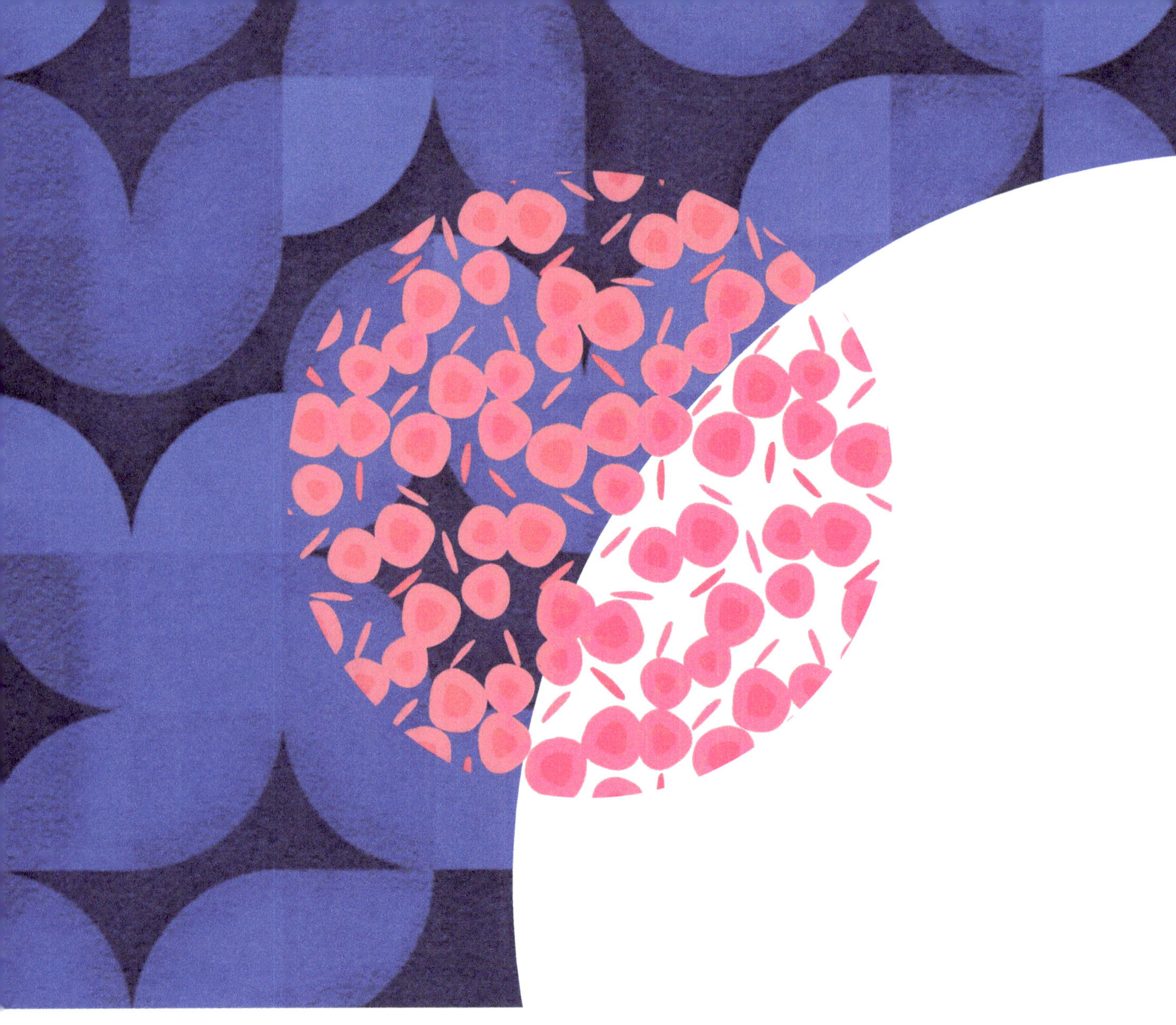

SCIENCE SIMPLIFIED!

How do we heal? How long does it take? Well, humans are pretty amazing. But we're not perfect. After you have surgery, things never go back to 100 percent, and we aren't just talking about the scars you can see.

During surgery, your body starts the work, which looks mostly like, "Stop the bleeding." This damage sets off a firestorm of gossip on the cellular level. Everyone starts talking, the phones light up, orders are placed, and the bossy cells start barking commands. It's like trying to make a Thanksgiving turkey for your extended family at your mother-in-law's house, and in the end, it all turns out great, but boy, can the process be painful! So, before I prompted the flashbacks of your last family gathering, I was talking about bleeding.

I hear you loud and clear! Sending in the troops!
Great! We have a lot of work to do!

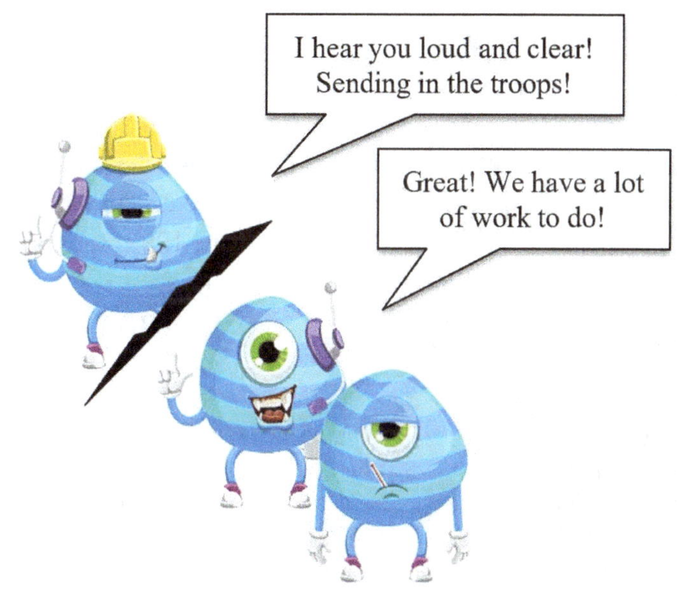

It starts with controlling the bleeding and alerting the body that there has been damage. That damage needs to be repaired, and fast! At about twenty-four hours, your skin has formed a pretty good seal to wall off the outside world, so you will be cleared to shower a day or two after surgery. As your body repairs the deeper layers over the next three weeks, the wound continues to strengthen. But things aren't considered "done" healing for up to two years. This depends on you and any healing issues you might have. And when I say healing issues, that includes radiation.

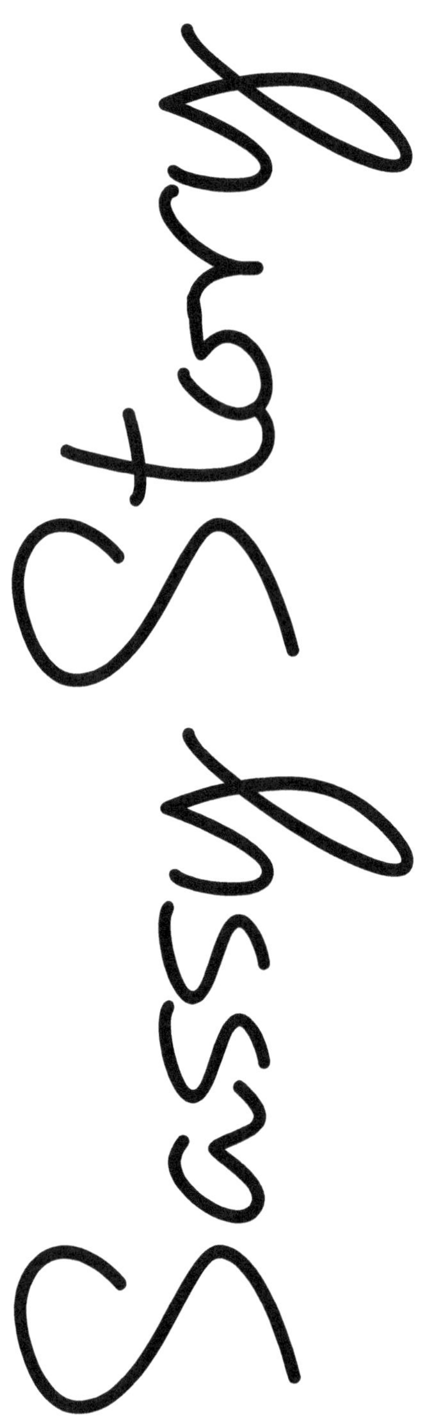

The history of breast cancer is not for the faint of heart. And you are definitely going through enough without thinking of these gruesome details. Suffice it to say, breast cancer is one of the oldest documented diseases. For the past several thousand years, every major civilization with a written language documented some account of breast cancer. They also took a literal "stab" at treating it. Unfortunately, those women were not as lucky as you are. (Yes, I said it—lucky.) These ladies didn't have the benefit of anesthesia (ouch!) or aseptic technique (germs, ew!), and the idea of bloodletting was popular for quite a long, long, long time. Anesthesia was first used in 1846, and the concept of the sterile technique wasn't championed until 1867. Let that information sink in! And for those of you who have the much-hated drainage tubes placed at the time of mastectomy or axillary lymph node dissection, those suckers first came about in 1858.

Since the dawn of "let's see if we can cut that off" several thousand years ago and on to 1882, things did not change much. And even then, with a standard "radical mastectomy" championed by Dr. Halstead, things were pretty . . . well—intense. We have scaled things way back in the surgical world. In 1882, when things were finally standardized for the first time, everyone who came in with a breast lump had everything but the rib cage removed. Sorry to the squeamish ladies out there! We are talking, breast, skin, pectoral muscles (major and minor), all the lymph nodes under the arm, and sometimes even the lymph nodes in the chest/neck/ clavicle area. Yikes! And that led to quite a significant amount of side effects (not to mention deaths). But, every science starts somewhere, and I think it's important to realize just how far we have come. Let's be grateful for the lessons learned from those who went before us and continually strive for improvement. Let's face it; we are still on a significant upswing toward better.

The next great evolution was in 1948 with the standardization of the modified radical mastectomy (abbreviated as MRM), which is the removal of the breast and lymph nodes under the arm. It is still performed today for those ladies undergoing mastectomy with positive lymph nodes. The chest wall muscles are left alone, and enough skin is left to close the wound. (Amen to that!)

And for all you ladies who aren't in the mastectomy camp, the advent of breast conservation finally arrived on the scene (in conjunction with radiation). While there were some accounts of lumpectomy being performed by some surgeons as early as the 1950s, the National Cancer Institute in the USA didn't endorse breast conservation until 1991. Like most significant changes in medicine, it took several large clinical trials in the US and abroad to prove the safety of lumpectomy. Yep, we are not that far away from some major changes in breast cancer management.

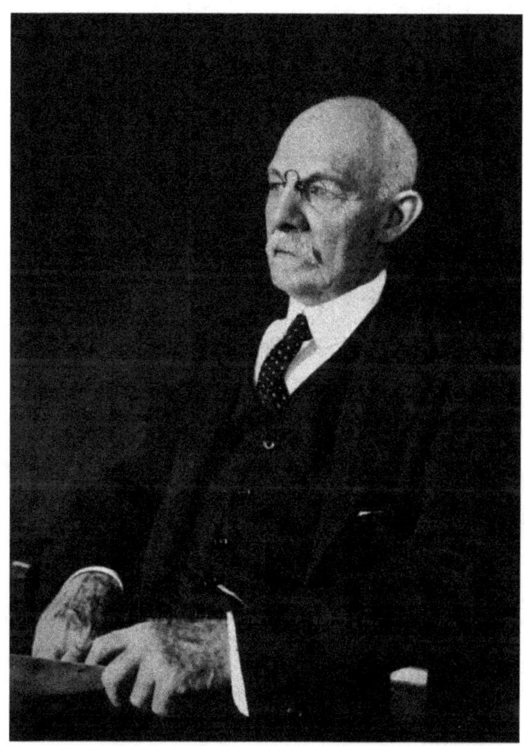

William Halstead, MD

And after reading the lymphedema section, you may indeed be surprised to realize that sentinel lymph nodes only became standard practice for women in 1994. Yes, less than thirty years ago you said goodbye to the whole island of lymph nodes and saw an upwards of 30 percent chance of lymphedema. Wowzah! Special shout-out to some fantastic surgical pioneers.

FAQS:

Frequently Asked Questions

Q. What if I am getting a lumpectomy and the surgeon "gets in there" and realizes that the cancer is bigger than expected? Could I wake up with a mastectomy?

A. Pretty much any breast surgeon will say no to this. Remember, surgeons don't know what's going on at the cellular level on the day of surgery anyway. But it's always important to talk with your surgeon about these fears. It is important to know that mastectomy could be discussed at your follow-up visit if you have multiple, unexpected positive margins. But we don't make this kind of "game day" decision.

Q. Is cancer going to spread when it "hits the air?"

A. This one's an old wives' tale. If you chose to believe it, then what are your options now? Leave the cancer where it is? Nope. Move on!

Q. Can I do anything to prevent lymphedema?

A. Yes, get yourself to physical therapy! And maybe, pending further study, some super-fancy surgery can prevent lymphedema (called a lymphovenous bypass).

Q. How many lymph nodes do I have?

A. We all have somewhere between a few and over sixty. We are all made differently, so the total number we each have doesn't mean much in the grand scheme of things.

Q. Why is my upper inner arm numb?

A. This is pretty common after lymph node surgery. The nerve that gives this area sensation runs right through the axillary (armpit) surgery spot. It's a small nerve that isn't easily seen, so it usually ends up cut. If you feel like you have a football under your arm and things feel odd, you aren't alone, and your body will find its new normal.

The BIG Day! Let's Get That Beastie Out!

Holy crap! For those of you who have had the honor of already enduring a handful of surgeries, this may seem like small beans. But for those of you who are surgery newbies . . . holy crap, right? All this lead-up, the anxiety, the waiting . . . and now you're going under the knife! And here it comes—the flood of panic. You are stricken with a case of the "what-ifs." What if I die? Sorry, sister, this is not likely to be your ticket to the next plane of existence. Your chance of dying in the next thirty days is less than 0.1 percent, regardless of which procedure you have. "But what if _____ ?" What if _____ ?" "What if the most horrible thing that a surgeon can image happens?" Eesh, don't you know that surgeons have been around the block? A lot of them have had some pretty dramatic waking nightmares or have at least heard of something happening once upon a time. Want the good news? The fantastical surgery stories that are the water-cooler talk for these knife-wielding ninjas are not about breast surgery. Sorry, little lady, breast surgery is not the "cool" Grey's Anatomy episode-worthy drama. In the grand scheme of surgeries, we are talking about some low-risk business.

Most breast surgeons don't devote their life to breast cancer because of the adrenaline rush. Naw! It's much more fun than that; it's for you, sweet lady! And it's for all the ladies who cannot decide between mastectomy and lumpectomy, or come in shaking with anxiety. It's because we love those quirky gals. Coincidentally, all this mushy talk usually makes the adrenaline junky surgeons want to chew their scrub caps. All right, the insight into the abyss is over. Take all those "what ifs" and kick them to the curb! Here's how a typical day before and day of surgery is going to go:

Day Before:

You may be asked to shower with some hospital-grade soap. After midnight, no food and no drinking (generally). This means that you should have a good meal and laugh with friends and family over a glass of wine (or whatever beverage strikes your fancy). Tomorrow is going to happen, and dwelling on the future doesn't call forth the moment any quicker. Please note, I did not say drink a bottle of wine and eat a Big Mac at 11:00 p.m. Listen, rabble-rouser, if you violate this rule, you should own up to it. You possibly might be looking at rescheduling your surgery. If you don't own up to it, you could be looking at some bad-news pneumonia. Anesthesiologists don't get any joy in starving people. Still, they do like a no-nonsense, no-complication procedure. An empty stomach is one step closer to a quick, uncomplicated nap!

Morning Of:

Show up on time or a little early. Our schedules are near impossible to predict. Life happens, stuff happens. Whatever time you were given is a rough estimate. Roll with it!

Pre-Op:

You are going to meet a lot of people. Don't worry, they don't bite. But they will poke you with sharp objects. (IVs may, in fact, be the most uncomfortable part of this whole shebang for some of you.)

You are going strip down to your birthday suit, put your clothes in a bag, get in a gown, and hop on a hospital stretcher. (Yikes! This is getting real!) Now, madam, you will start your receiving line: nurses to start IVs, nurses that will be in the OR, nurses that will be assisting in the OR, nurses that are giving a break to the nurse that poked you, your surgeon, and your anesthesiologist. And there's going to be paperwork. Signatures. You will be asked, "What are you having done today?" by so many people that it may begin to sound funny. Like the time you said a word over and over until it lost all meaning. You sign so much paperwork that you may be surprised to learn that you have not, in fact, purchased a house by the end of all of it.

Your surgeon will draw a big yes on the correct side . . . or maybe both sides (which in retrospect may seem a bit like overkill).

You are going to be told a whole lotta stuff that you are definitely not going to remember. (The memory thing is not entirely the fault of your anxiety. You can put some blame on "retrograde amnesia" from that drug-toting anesthesiologist.)

Kiss your family and friends and relegate them to an uncomfortable waiting room chair and hospital food. Off you go! Whoosh!

The OR:

When you are finally wheeled to the OR, you will meet the "pit crew," and you may well feel like a race car coming in for a pit stop! You've got an anesthesiologist and possibly a certified registered nurse anesthetist to assist during the procedure. You also have a circulating nurse who will be managing the room while everyone else is "sterile" in their gown and gloves, a scrub tech who hands stuff to the surgeons. (Yes, it's soooo cool—just like the movies. It's also very hard to turn off when at home assembling furniture or changing lightbulbs!) Don't forget the surgeon and possibly an extra scrub tech or "first assistant," who acts as the surgeon's third and fourth hands because (sometimes) two is not enough. If you are at an academic institution, these extra hands are likely residents in training or medical students. Do not fear the doctor in training; your doctor was there once, and it was through the gifts of prior patients that you are able to trust them with your life now. Let those young people observe or help; they are under strict supervision and have to earn participation. You may also have a medical device rep if your surgeon is using some new gear. And finally, a radiology tech may come in to take an X-ray of what you just said "goodbye" to, and another person will come to collect the specimen to run it to pathology. See? It's a pit crew!

You will be asked to move yourself to the OR table (yes, it's narrow!). Nurses will start putting massaging booties on your calves (these prevent blood clots). Warm blankets come next because those ORs are damn cold! The

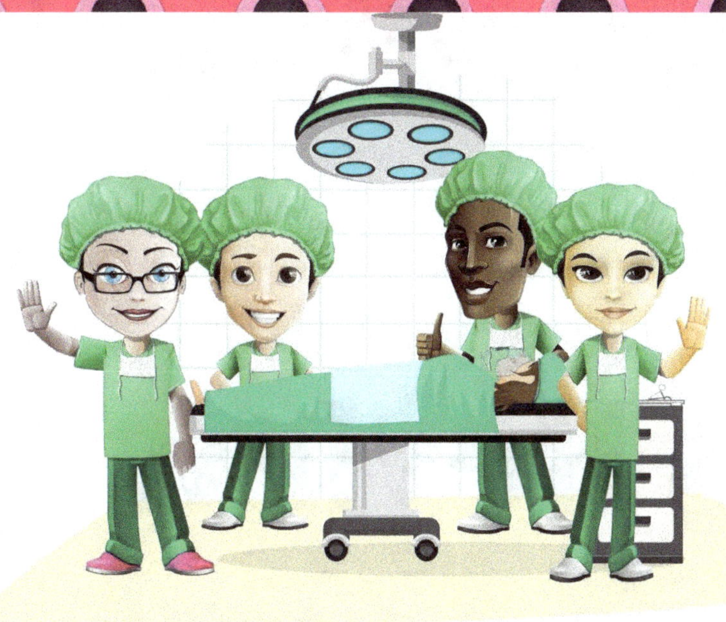

anesthesiologist will put on stickers (ECG leads, BIS monitor), a blood pressure cuff (which will get so terribly tight the first time), a pulse oximeter, and a mask with oxygen (which smells like a plastic beach ball). They will warn you that your IV may burn a little, then ask you to count back from ten . . . nine . . . eight.

You will get your surgery—bada-bing, bada-boom. The best part: you won't remember any of this.

PACU (AKA Post-Anesthesia Recovery Unit):

You will wake up in the post-anesthesia recovery area (PACU). Note that it is to recover from the anesthesia (because we all know that recovery from the surgery takes days, not hours).

A PACU recovery nurse will make sure you have something to eat and drink and keep your pain manageable. Manageable means that you can move and take deep breaths. If you sit like a statue and try to be stoic, you will end up with pneumonia and blood clots, so knock it off, Joan of Arc. If you are going home, they will usually make sure you urinate, go over discharge instructions, and get you in a wheelchair to the curb for pickup. Or they will bid you adieu on your way to a hospital room. See? Easy peasy!

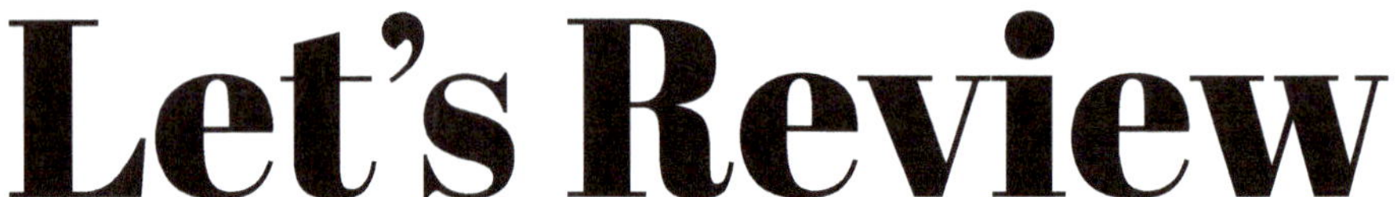

Let's Review

- You may not be a candidate for surgery if you have significant health problems.

- You may not be a candidate for breast conservation (keeping your breast and removing only the cancer).

- If you are a candidate for mastectomy and lumpectomy (lumpectomy is almost always coupled with radiation), there is no survival advantage to mastectomy (unless you are a pathogenic genetic variant carrier). That means that you will not live longer if you chose mastectomy.

- Lumpectomy almost always means radiation. Mastectomy sometimes means radiation.

- You may need to return to the operating room if there is cancer at the cut edge.

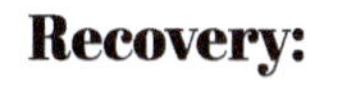

Recovery:

- Lumpectomy: Two weeks (no drains)

- Mastectomy: Four weeks (yes, drains)

- Mastectomy with reconstruction: Six weeks (yes, drains)

- You are lawfully entitled to breast reconstruction after mastectomy. Reconstruction can be started at the time of mastectomy or at any time after (one, five, or even ten years afterward, as long as you are healthy enough for surgery).

- If there is no evidence of cancer in the lymph nodes under your arm (in your armpit), the surgeon may sample the nodes under your arm at the time of your breast surgery.

- If you are found to have cancer in the lymph nodes under your arm, you may be offered removal of all the nodes under your arm.

- Removal of lymph nodes under the arm carries a risk of arm swelling called lymphedema.

Words from Your Sisters:

You are not alone!

Radiation was the worst part of the whole thing! I burned and blistered!

Survivor Sister

I almost didn't get radiation after what my dad went through with prostate cancer radiation; but, in the end, it really wasn't that bad.

Survivor Sister

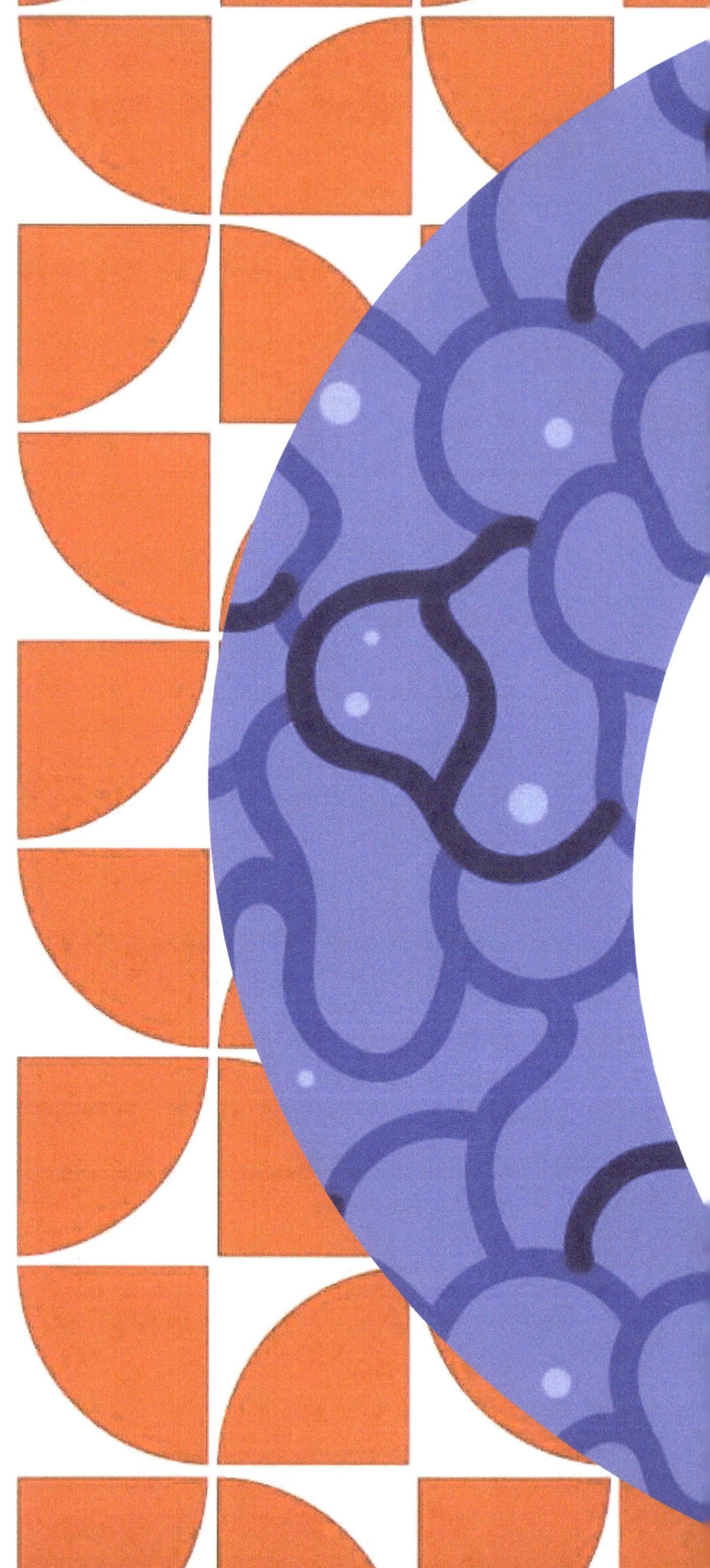

Radiation

A Day at the Beach

Remember the last time you read the warning label on your standard store-bought pain reliever? Yeah, me neither. So remember, as you navigate adjuvant therapies (the doctor word for the treatments that aren't surgery), that everything in life has side effects (heck, eating lettuce or cookie dough carries the risk of death from E.coli or salmonella). Keep in mind that whenever we talk about treatment options, we weigh risks and benefits. For some, the risk will be higher than the benefit and vice versa. As always, (broken record, I know!) listen to your doctor, they are your partner in crime and are there to help you understand the risks and benefits to you! Disclaimer aside, here's the lowdown on the "day at the beach." (Yes, it's a bad joke. But where else do you end up with a skin burn and that "I spent all day laying in the sun" fatigue?)

Now, if you are one of those unfortunate ladies who has known someone who has had radiation, you may be saying "No, no, no." But I beg you to keep an open mind. Breast radiation is vastly different from pelvic or head and neck radiation (those can certainly be bad business). Because let's face it, the head, neck, and pelvis each have super-essential life functions (like eating, swallowing, talking, urinating, and defecating). Breasts, thankfully, do not.

What Is Radiation?

Zap!

Um, Sweetie… I think you might have had enough sun for today.

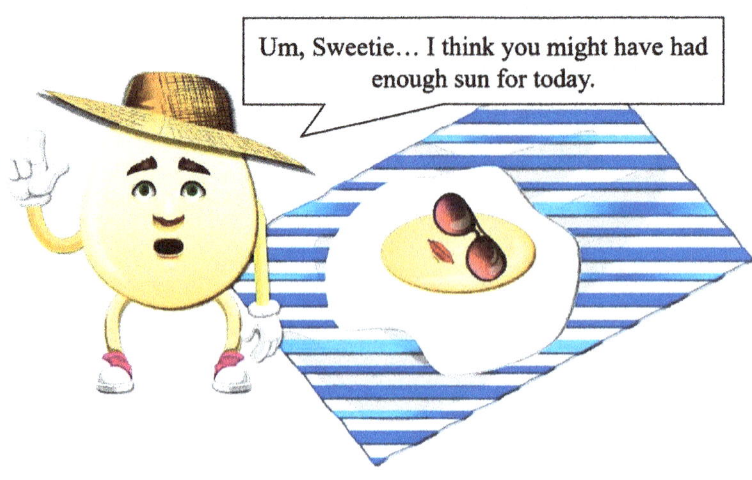

Radiation is energy, and no, it's not the "I don't want to get out of bed today" kind of energy. It's the type of energy produced by radioactive materials or machines called linear accelerators. And this type of energy cannot be seen or felt.

How does radiation work? We are back to the cookies and the recipe—again. Radiation rips up the recipe (it makes small breaks in the DNA). Cells that are dividing fast (like cancer cells) just cannot paste the recipe back together fast enough to make new cookies; therefore they die. As a result, the cookies (cancer cells) stop getting made. Nearby normal cells also sustain little rips in their recipe, but they aren't trying to use the recipe to divide quickly, and they have some time to sit and put the DNA recipe back together.

Radiation is not for every breast cancer patient. But there are certainly many women for whom radiation is recommended. (Think about it: all lumpectomy ladies and some ladies after mastectomy who have big cancers, cancers that spread to the lymph nodes, as well as some other features that we find out from the pathologists.)

Lumpectomy ladies, you need radiation. Period. End of story. (Okay, there are a few exceptions.)

Wait! Slow your roll, docs! My surgeon is going to remove all the cancer from my breast, so why isn't that enough? Sorry, sister, but as effective as surgery is, one of its best friends is radiation. They are both for local treatment (meaning that they both treat the breast and sometimes the lymph nodes, period). Again, I must repeat: they are local treatment—just for the breast and lymph nodes. They do not treat the body (that is for chemotherapy, which is why you cannot get out of chemo because you do more surgery or radiation). Radiation does not extend its reach beyond the breast. It does not cause hair loss. Interestingly, to your advantage, there is a caveat here called the abscopal effect (see the "science simplified" section on page 104). A good way to think about radiation is the lawn analogy. (Oh yay, I just love a good analogy and, as promised, more gardening analogies.)

Suppose you have a beautiful green lawn with a giant weed in the middle. That weed is the cancer. We see it on imaging or feel it. The surgeon is the gardener who pulls that weed. Ta-da! Weed-free lawn, right? But we all know what happens the next time it rains. More weeds. To prevent these weeds (what would be a cancer recurrence), we need to spray that lawn with weed treatment. That weed treatment is the radiation. Radiation cuts the chance of you getting cancer back in that breast (a recurrence) by about half (or more).

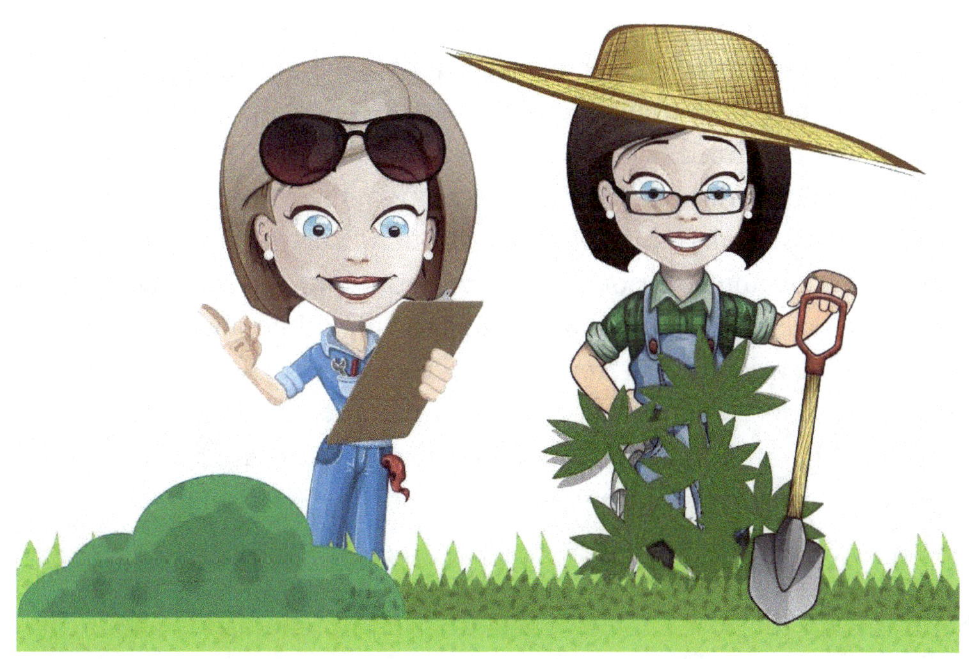

Radiation Oncologist: "*Looks like I am here to spray the lawn!*"
Surgeon: "*I just need to pull this weed out first and then I'll get out of your way!*"

Mastectomy ladies, the same lawn principle applies to you if you check one of the boxes for "post-mastectomy radiation." Surgery removed the cancer. But due to the features of your cancer, the lawn that is left (the skin and small amounts of breast cells attached to that skin) needs some weed treatment and TLC (tender-loving-care).

Radiation comes in several flavors. Here is when you tune into your doctor's expert opinion. Please, please (I beg you), do not pull out this page and try to "teach" your doc or argue with your doc. If you don't trust your doc to make the right decision with you, then you need a new doc. Here's a brief rundown of what you may be offered and the side effects. Keep in mind that not every hospital has each of these options. And that's okay! Each of these options has stringent criteria, and you certainly may not be a candidate for some of these therapies.

External Beam Radiation

WBI or "whole breast irradiation"—the "tried and true" old Bessie—none of that new fandangled stuff. However, not wanting to sell modern-day WBI short, there have been tremendous changes to how WBI is performed, and it's much more refined than it was several decades ago! If you think back to the lawn analogy, this one fits nicely. You treat the whole lawn for up to seven weeks every darn day, Monday through Friday. You will go in for some longer planning sessions (about an hour each), get some fancy tattoos (okay, they aren't really anything to go showing off because they really just look like oddly dark, small freckles), and then you are set for the daily session that lasts about ten to fifteen minutes. The actual treatment only lasts a couple of minutes (think of it as a long X-ray; you don't see or feel anything), and you can drive yourself home.

Chest wall irradiation or post-mastectomy radiation is the same idea as WBI, but this is for the post-mastectomy ladies who need radiation. Your chest wall or reconstructed breast will get a long X-ray every day for up to seven weeks.

Also, if your cancer beasties made it to your lymph nodes, the remaining nodes that drain the breast could get a zap too! These are lymph nodes remaining under the arm, around the collar bone, and sometimes the lymph nodes hanging out behind your sternum. Not everyone needs this therapy, and we will leave that to the experts.

External beam radiation can take three main forms, delivered by electrons, photons, or protons. Dr. David Schomas gives a breakdown of proton therapy in the "Expert Extras" chapter at the end of the book on page 190. Take a look-see.

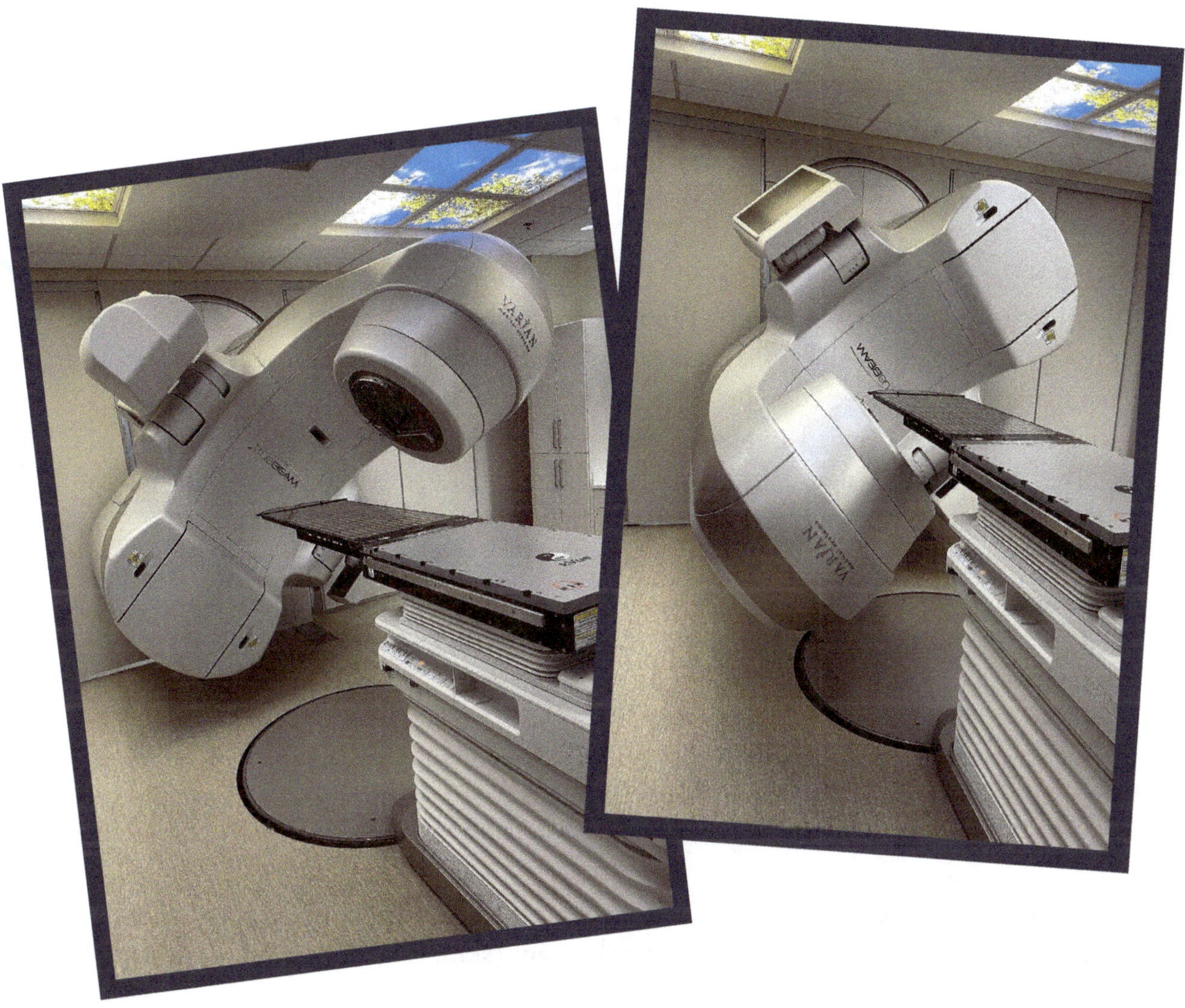

Linear Accelerator

Photos courtesy of Astrid Morrison, MD

Brachytherapy or Internal Radiation "What Is It?"

by Astrid Morrison, M.D.

Brachytherapy is delivered using one or more radioactive sources (typically about the size of a grain of rice) inserted into the breast using one or multiple catheters. Brachy comes from the Greek word, which means "short," meaning that the radiation is given off at short distances. The most commonly used form of brachytherapy for breast cancer is high dose-rate brachytherapy (HDR), which means the radiation is given off very quickly by the radioactive source, so the treatment only takes a matter of minutes. This is in contrast to low-dose rate brachytherapy, which takes days or sometimes even months to deliver the full dose.

HDR brachytherapy is administered using a radiation device called a remote afterloader (pictured to the right). The radioactive source is housed inside it and is on the end of a long wire about the diameter of fishing line. It is sent through the transfer tubes, which are connected to the catheters in the breast down into the breast tissue, where it spends a specified amount of time based upon computer calculations to deliver the prescribed amount of radiation to the breast tissue immediately around the lumpectomy site. Another term for this method of radiation is partial breast irradiation (PBI). In order to be treated with HDR brachytherapy, a woman must undergo placement of a device into the breast, such as the SAVI (Strut Adjusted Volume Implant) device shown to the right, several weeks after the initial lumpectomy.

Some women are better candidates for HDR brachytherapy using multiple catheters that are placed around the lumpectomy cavity (pictured to the right), for example, most women with breast implants.

There are advantages of PBI over WBI: shorter course of treatment (ten treatments over five days) and less radiation to normal organs (skin, ribs, lung, heart). But not all women are candidates for PBI.

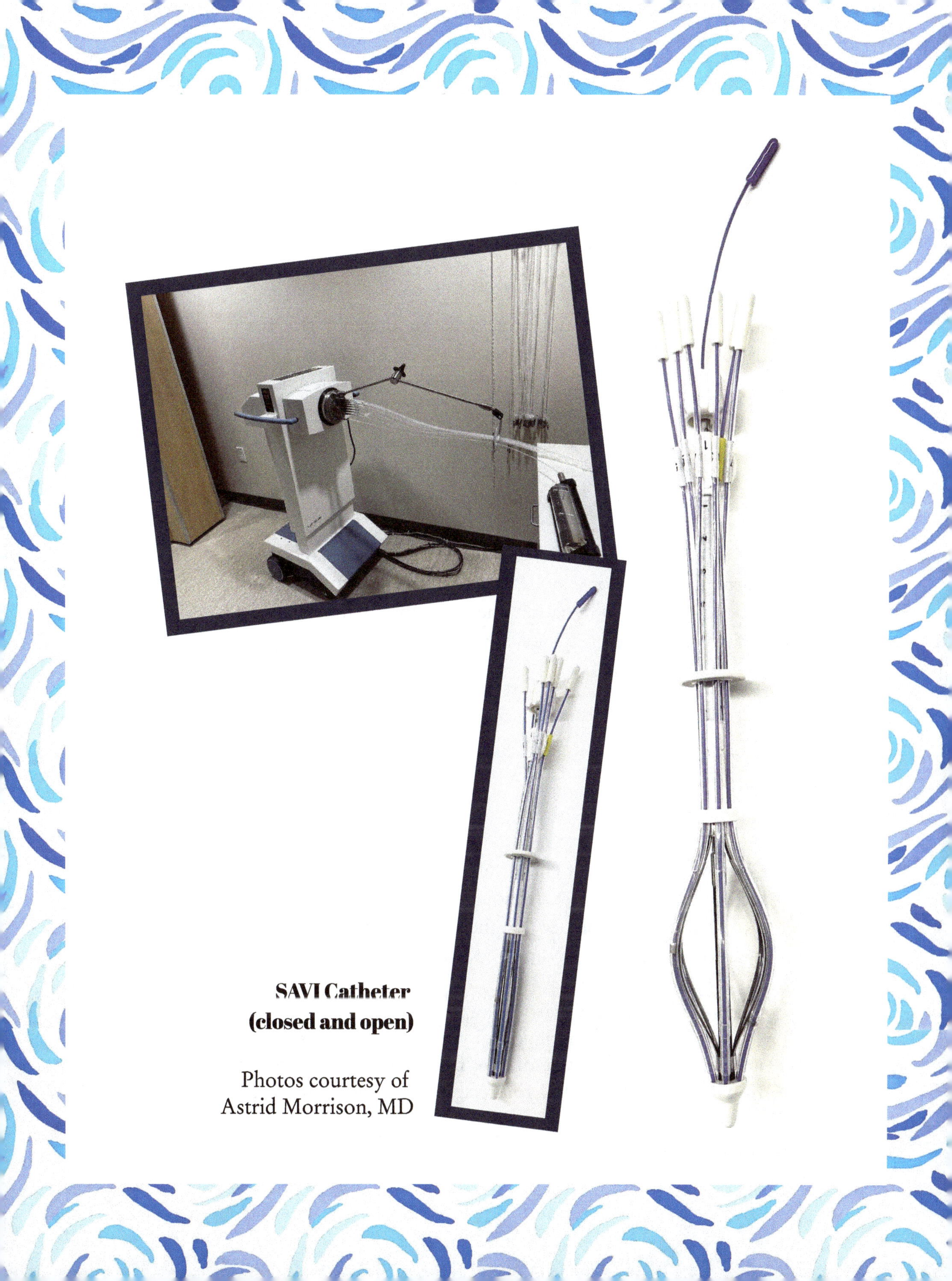

SAVI Catheter (closed and open)

Photos courtesy of Astrid Morrison, MD

Thank you, Dr. Morrison! In summary, you may be offered a return trip to the OR for insertion of a temporary device. This device allows you to get targeted radiation to the lumpectomy site. You and your doctor will have to decide if you are a candidate for this therapy. Keep in mind that it will often require an extra procedure (to place the device) but overall fewer days of driving into the hospital for radiation.

Moving on to IORT, or intra-operative radiation therapy: This is a single dose of radiation given while you are asleep, at the time of surgery, by a radiation device placed right into your breast, where the cancer was, right after your cancer is removed. IORT is an investigational treatment and is certainly not available at every institution in the country. Some specific criteria need to be met to qualify for this treatment as it continues to be studied.

This is certainly not an all-inclusive rundown on all things radiation that are currently offered or may be offered in the near future. If you are offered another type of radiation, then tune into that brilliant radiation oncologist. They may be tailoring your care to your specific scenario. One size does not fit all!

Radiation Side Effects

Enter All the Scary Possibilities . . .

- You will have a lower chance of your breast cancer coming back! What a great effect. Although it's not an actual side effect, it's an important reminder that the stuff that follows is generally regarded as small beans compared to getting your cancer back.

- Fatigue. This usually starts a couple of weeks into therapy, and for most is akin to the fatigue that you have after a long day outside. It might slow you down a bit, but it doesn't keep you from doing the things that you really want to do. Also, in case you need another excuse to get active, exercise, such as walking for twenty minutes three to four times a week can help tremendously.

• Skin changes. This is likened to a sunburn without the fun of laying poolside. During therapy, you will be asked to slather on a ton of lotions, oils, and ointments two to three times daily (but not within two hours of starting treatment). You may never have a skin problem, or you may get something like the worst sunburn you can imagine with red, peeling skin (it's temporary!). Afterward, you may end up with skin that is darker than the rest of you. Everyone is different. Only time will tell.

That's it! These are the big ones. There are many more in the fine print, but the chances that they will affect you are small.

• Inflammation in the lung. This happens in about 2 percent of ladies (rare!) and shows up one to six months after you finish radiation. The symptoms are usually mild and go away on their own. You could have a dry cough, low-grade fever, shortness of breath, chest pain, and/or fatigue. Rarely, steroids may be needed.

• Scarring of the lung. We aren't talkin' the kind of scarring that you would notice the next time you go on a run. It's basically like an "internal scar" or just some marks on your lung that a radiologist would see on a CT scan if you ever needed one in the future. It's certainly far less damaging than smoking cigarettes.

• Damage to the heart. This is only a concern for left-sided cancers, since your heart is under your left breast. But the effects are far less significant on your heart than, say, smoking or eating unhealthy foods and not working out. There are also techniques to minimize this damage (like breath-holding techniques to get your lungs to push your heart farther away from the chest wall). With modern radiation approaches and techniques, risks to your heart are very minimal, if any at all.

- And there's always the small chance of radiation causing another cancer . . . "Wait, what? Hold the phone. Are you kidding me? There's a curse planted in the cure?" Well, yes and no. Has it happened? Yes. But this risk is much, much much smaller than the risk of getting breast cancer again if you don't get the radiation. The very rare event of a cancer caused by radiation therapy is approximately 1 in 50,000 in ten to twenty years. Like many health problems, it's multifactorial (which is medical jargon for "it's a problem caused by more than one thing"). For example, think about how heart disease is caused by genes, smoking, diet, and exercise. Getting another cancer from radiation can be impacted by many factors—especially smoking. Have we mentioned that smoking is bad for you? Risks and benefits, right?

- Damage to any and all nearby structures . . . yeah, it doesn't sound good. Radiation hits anything near the breast, at least a little bit. We have covered the big ones (heart and lungs), but radiation can also affect your ribs and make them more prone to breaking if you have some future trauma.

Take a deep breath. I know, this is just the pits! But we can do this! And remember, even the package insert for over-the-counter medications can include . . . death. Life is not without side effects. Surgery has side effects, but we need to get that cancer out! Radiation has side effects, but for some women, it will be the difference between a cancer-free future and having to go through this whole thing again. Breathe. Take a big deep breath. You'll get through this one step at a time.

Heart Disease and Radiation

by David Schomas, M.D

This subject has gotten lots of attention over the past few years. Maybe too much. In the past, we looked around and saw women with heart disease who had radiation for their left-sided breast cancer. The heart is on the left side of the chest. Therefore, radiation to the left breast caused heart disease. Case closed, right?

Not so fast, my friend. As I sit here typing these words into my laptop, enjoying a lukewarm Americano, I look out the window and watch the rain fall. People are running around with their umbrellas. Come to think of it, every time it rains, I see umbrellas out. That must mean that umbrellas cause the rain. Case closed, right?

The reality is always more complicated. Think of heart disease as a recipe for disease—not a fun recipe for chili on a cold, rainy day. To make chili, it takes many ingredients in the right amounts. Then it needs to be heated, slow cooked, and simmered, right? Just like you cannot make chili with one or two ingredients, you cannot make heart disease with only radiation. It takes a number of factors: family history, genetics, cholesterol levels, exercise, weight, blood pressure, stress, fitness, diet, age, previous chemotherapy, and yes, maybe even radiation therapy—especially if the radiation is not designed and delivered properly with the proper modern techniques. The good news? We do have proper modern techniques.

All right, curious cats . . .

Radiation is some real science. It's super complex, so a couple of paragraphs are just not going to cut it here. That said, here we go . . . Remember, radiation rips up our cookie recipe, which means that it makes small breaks in the DNA, but this only happens to the cells that are exposed. This is a local effect; the radiation has to hit the actual cells to affect them. This means that the cells that aren't in the vicinity of the breast are not affected.

Cells that are dividing fast, like cancer cells, can't paste the recipe back together fast enough to make new cookies; therefore they die. Ta-da! Dead cancer cells. Nearby normal cells also sustain little rips in their recipe, but they aren't trying to use the recipe to divide quickly (make more cookies), and they have some time to put the DNA recipe back

SCIENCE SIMPLIFIED!

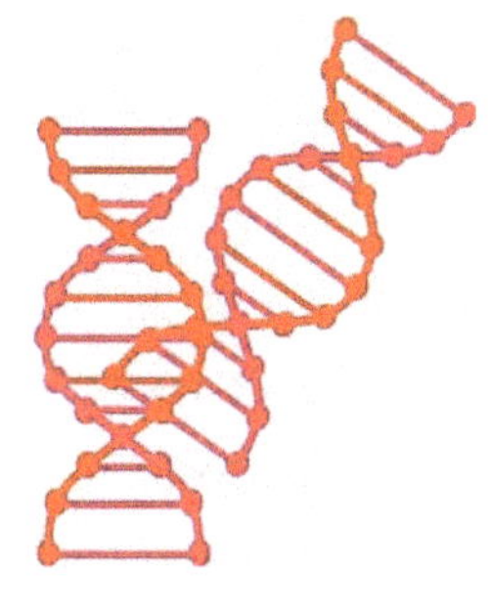

together. When these cells don't put the DNA recipe back the exact right way, they can keep those mistakes in their recipe and (very rarely) make new cancer.

Okay, let's start at the cellular level. Imagine the DNA double helix (or see the picture above), the literal instruction manual to build life; it is minding its own business (or potentially in the act of copying itself), when all the of a sudden energy rays (X-rays, gamma-rays, and free radicals) start riddling the DNA with breaks. No more recipe; no more cancer cells.

All right, you're likely thinking, I got it, now what on earth is actually making this radiation? And how? What on earth is happening in that large machine (the linear accelerator) that I am lying down under for external beam radiation? And all I can say is "science magic." This is some crazy science magic. May I suggest searching the internet for "how does a linear particle accelerator work?" It is impressive and complex and way too complicated to simplify here. There are electrons, electron guns, radiofrequency waves, waveguides, magnets called steering targets, tungsten, copper, water, digital accelerators, vacuums, and collimators. All of these make a beam of X-rays (photons) that come out in a highly planned and measured way. Bam! Zap!

As promised, we will also touch on what is called the abscopal effect. This will sound like some crazy, wondrous stuff, and it is still debated to this day. In the 1950s, a radiobiologist R.H. Mole observed treatment-related changes outside of the radiation field. Unpacked, this means that radiation applied to a tumor in one area of the body seemed to make other tumors or metastatic tumors outside of the radiation field also shrink. How? We just said radiation is local; it doesn't have any effect on the tissues outside of the zapper beam. Enter the debate. This effect has been observed in several types of cancers. The simplified gist is that radiation to one tumor starts killing the beastie cancers at that location. This alerts the immune system to these baddies. The immune system then gets ramped up and goes out into the body looking for more baddies. The immune system starts fighting and killing cancer outside of the radiation field. Now, the extent of this within a single person is hard to quantify. Suffice it to say, radiation has some significant benefits.

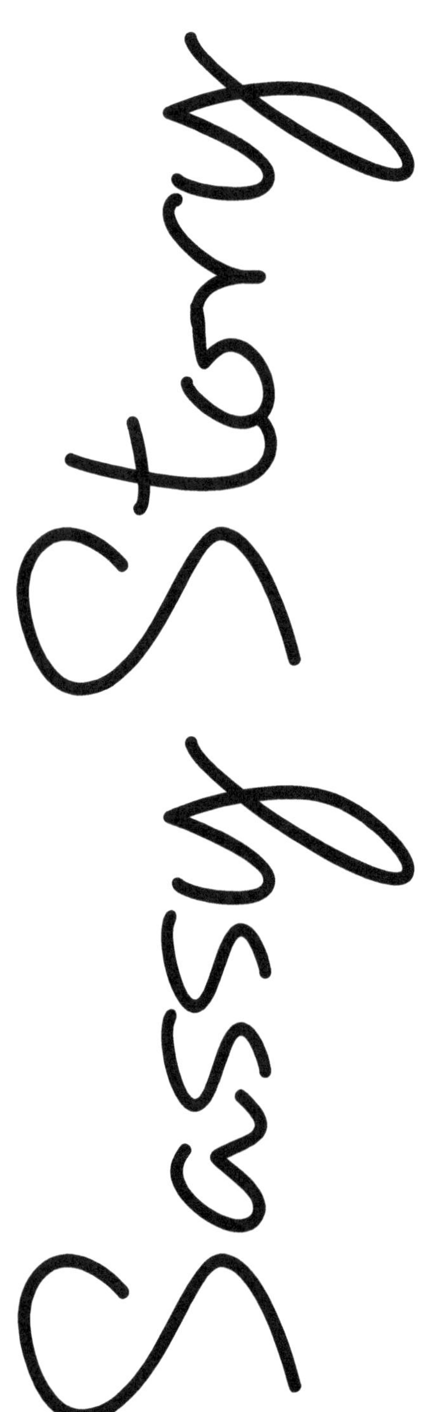

We already know that Wilhelm Conrad Röntgen discovered X-rays in 1895. This set off a whirlwind of discoveries in the field that eventually became what we have today through some science, blood, sweat, and tears. Radiation oncology (the use of radiation to treat cancer) had a humble start; not more than two weeks after the discovery of radiation, a medical student in Chicago, Emil Herman Grubbe, tried to treat cancer for the first time. And what cancer might that have been? Yep! Breast cancer is a trailblazer again! Also, gee whiz, what a time! Medical students were running around with radiation, zapping people! Interestingly, this pioneering gentleman had to have ninety-two separate tumors removed due to his radiation exposure but still lived to the age of eighty-five.

Shortly thereafter, in 1898, Maria Sklodowska-Curie and her husband Pierre Curie discovered radium as a source of radiation. (They also discovered and named two new elements of the periodic table.) Three years later, the effects of radiation on humans was being published. In case you have not heard of this fierce lady, Marie Curie was the first person to win two Nobel Prizes, and she won them in two scientific fields. That is a huge deal! Nowadays, the unit of radioactivity of a radioisotope is still called a "curie!"

By the 1920s, radiation was mostly being used for skin cancers (since these were the easy-to-access cancers), and radiation oncologists started to realize that dividing exposure into several treatments lessened side effects (what we now call fractionated dosing). Radium-based brachytherapy was also used to treat deeper organs (gynecologic, head, and neck tumors). But even then, things were rudimentary at best. It was not until 1932 that docs even knew how much radiation they were giving (enter the ionizing chamber). From 1930–1950 a ton of changes were being made. Brachytherapy (internal radiation) was vastly improving, and external beam radiation therapy was born (external radiation capable of treating deep tumors). Between 1950–1980 more potent high energy rays, cobalt teletherapy, and later linear accelerators were becoming the norm. Hold up! If you are starting to skim and have flashbacks to high school history, just take a moment to realize that this is a significant change in a small amount of time. Also, please recognize that these discoveries allowed for the treatment of deeper tumors with less damage to the skin (yes, we certainly like that!). Also, an interesting fact, the invention of the nuclear reactor in the Manhatten Project during WWII paved the way for the creation of artificial radioisotopes for medical use in radiotherapy.

In the 1970s and 1980s, the much-buzzed-about proton therapy was introduced. Finally, by 1990 sophisticated computers were able to construct 3D treatment plans. Since then, things have continued to get more and more high-tech! As you can see, what started as a flamethrower, which unfortunately probably created more cancer than it cured, is now more like a sniper rifle (pew, pew!).

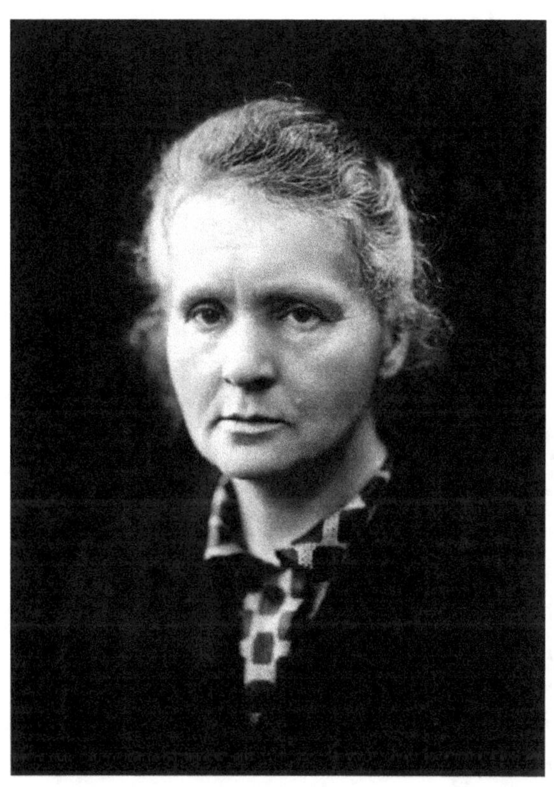

Marie Curie c. 1920

FAQS:

Frequently Asked Questions

Q. Will I lose my hair?

A. Not from radiation, sister. (Leave that bad business to the chemo.)

Q. Will my skin burn?

A. Yes and no. Everyone reacts differently! Remember a time when you stayed in the sun all day with your friends (possibly sipping on piña coladas)? Some of them turned beet red and blistered, and some turned a nice golden brown; we all react differently. In the same way that you should wear sunscreen in the sun to protect your skin, you will be asked to slather up with lotion or oil multiple times a day. Take note that this skincare should continue after your treatment finishes!

Q. Do I need proton therapy?

A. I think about it in terms of gardening again. You need loppers (those giant scissors) to trim a hedge, and you need a pair of small shears to prune a bonsai bush (those little miniature trees). Here, the loppers and the hedge are standard breast radiation and the breast. The small shears and the bonsai bush are proton therapy and cancer in some tight, high-stakes territory like the head (near the very important brain), the neck (needed to speak and swallow), or the pelvis (needed to go to the bathroom). You can undoubtedly prune a hedge with small shears ... you just don't need to. See Dr. David Schomas' expert opinion on page 190 for more details.

Q. Why do I need so many radiation treatments?

A. Like many things in life, think moderation. Let's imagine you buy a case of your favorite wine. You don't sit down and try to plow through the whole case in one sitting! You have a glass of wine every night with dinner. It's the same idea with radiation. A little bit every day is good. All of it at once . . . no! In the same way that your body needs time to process the alcohol before the next glass of wine, so, too, does the body need time to recover from the radiation before the next dose.

Q. How do we know the radiation therapy is working?

A. Well, we don't have a reliable way to measure if it's working because the tumor is gone, and there's nothing to monitor.

Q. Why did my doctor prescribe a boost?

A. A boost is a little bit of extra radiation right to the area where the tumor was, with the goal of decreasing recurrence. It is particularly effective in women under fifty years old with DCIS. But in the end, we will leave it up to those smart radiation oncologists to determine if you need a boost.

Q. Will I glow?

A. Sorry, no glowing like an alien and no glowing like a pregnant lady. While we are on the topic, you aren't radioactive, so you can snuggle up to as many pregnant ladies and babies as you'd like!

Q. I already had radiation. Can I have it again?

A. No, and yes. In general, the same breast doesn't get a second round of radiation (with rare exceptions). Body parts have a maximum safe amount of lifetime radiation. Period. If you had the left breast radiated in the past, you have a green light to radiate the right breast. But if your cancer has come back on the same side, you are likely looking at a mastectomy to avoid another round of radiation.

The BIG Day! Zap Me!

You show up, fill out some paperwork, and check-in. You have already had a chat with the radiation oncologist and decided what type of radiation they will be using. And it's whole-breast, external beam radiation. Tried and true.

Simulation Day

- You undress from the waist up and get into a gown that opens in the front.

- You are brought into the CT (or CAT) scanner room where you are laid on the CT scanner table and onto a bean bag or mold of sorts. This is *your* mold, fitted specific to you.

- Your arms go above your head, the breast in question is exposed, and the rest of you is covered.

- You get moved in and out of a CT scanner. While you are lying there, a radiation oncologist comes and checks the scan.

- They give the "go ahead," and laser beams shoot across the room. (Okay, the lasers are way less cool or noticeable than this sounds in writing.) The radiation therapist gives you little tattoos where those laser beams hit the skin. No, not a standard tattoo gun, just a tiny hospital-grade needle to inject some ink under the skin. Why the tattoo? In the future, your tattoos will be lined up with the lasers to make sure that you are in the exact right spot each time.

Planning session done! You'll get dressed and go home while the radiation oncologist and the dosimetrists plan and plan and plan.

Block Check Day

The next step is the dress rehearsal. You are going to come back one more time for a dry run. Same deal, no radiation yet. Just a check before all systems go! And then, the next time you come in, you show up for the real deal. You will schedule all your planned treatments, which are usually at the same time every day. Try your best not to miss treatments; however, you can adjust treatment times and makeup sessions for inclement weather and life events if necessary. Life is not always predictable!

Treatment Starts

Every single session will be the same!

You get on your mold. The lasers and tattoos align like star-crossed lovers and zip, zap, zoom for several minutes. You feel nothing, then drive yourself home. You will moisturize at home two to three times daily.

Rinse and repeat! And moisturize!

Let's Review

- Not everyone needs radiation.

- With very rare exception, everyone that gets a lumpectomy gets radiation.

- Some women will need radiation after mastectomy, but most will not.

- Radiation lowers your chance of recurrence and can increase your chance of survival.

- Nothing in life is without side effects, and radiation is no exception to this rule. The big ones are skin burn and fatigue.

- Radiation comes in multiple "flavors." Talk with your radiation oncologist to know what is right for you.

- Radiation can take as little as one week or as many as seven weeks.

Thoughts and Questions About Radiation

Words from Your Sisters:

You are not alone!

I lost my hair, but I never once looked at myself in the mirror without my wig on. The only people who saw me bald were the OR staff on the day of my surgery. They made sure it was back on when I woke up!

Survivor Sister

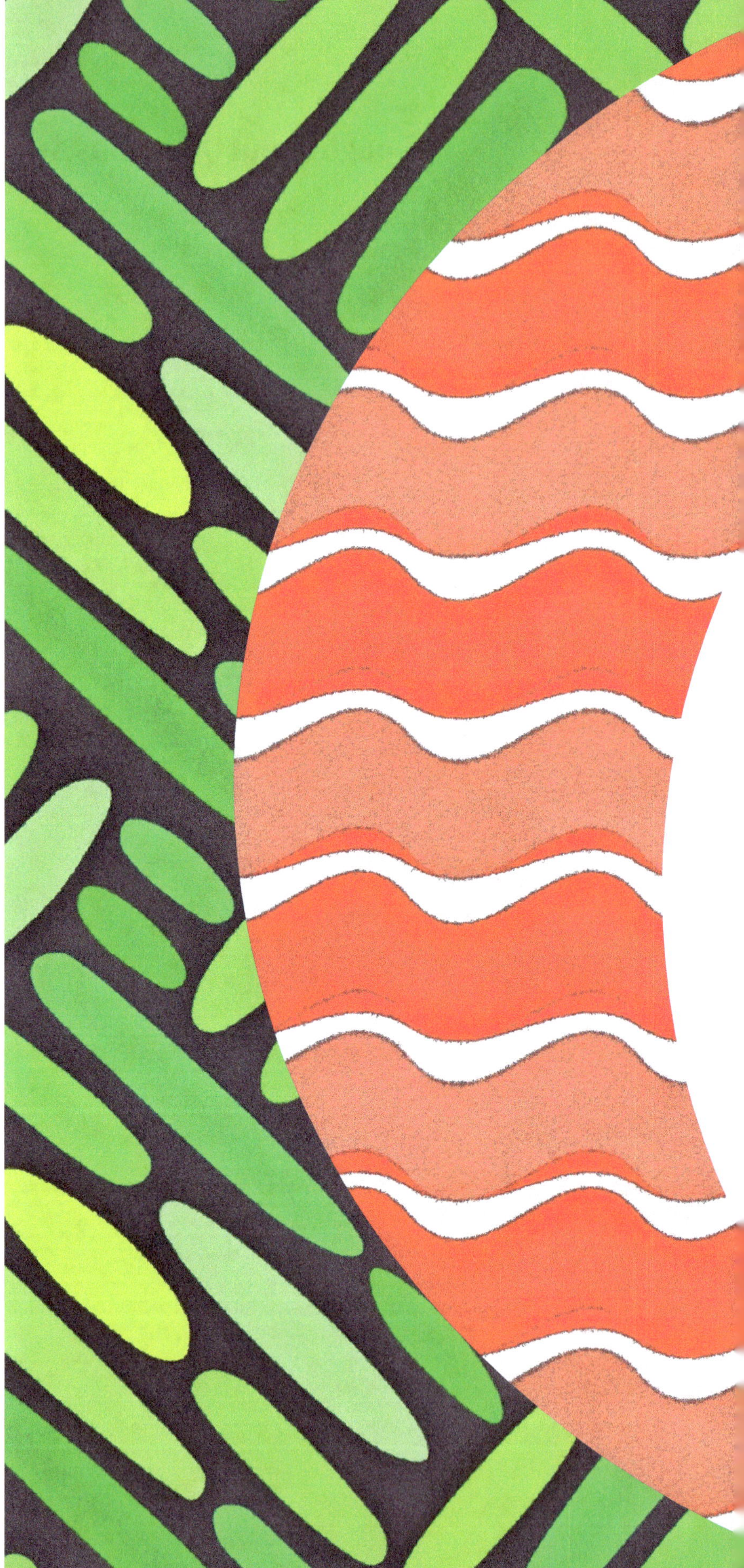

Medical Oncology

Bartender!

A medical oncologist is your best friend, bartender mixologist. They are going to see you regularly, listen to your problems, serve you up a cocktail (although not the one you want), and tailor your cocktail to your needs (cut you off when needed, give you a glass of water, and tell you when to walk it off).

Find someone you want to see . . . a lot . . . for several years. They will be in charge of chemotherapy, HER-2 receptor-targeted therapy, anti-estrogen pills, and any other innovative therapy options you may have access to through clinical trials.

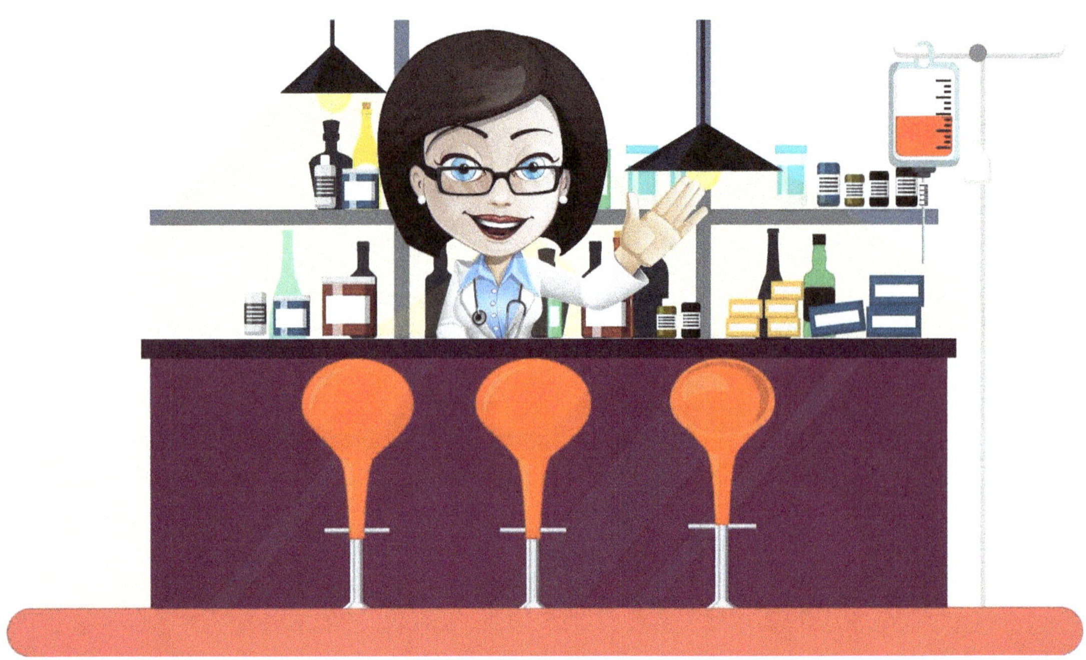

Estrogen and/or Progesterone Receptor-Positive

If you are negative for *both*—SKIP THIS! You have enough on your plate!

You will be asked to take a pill every day for five to ten years that blocks estrogen. So stop your hormone replacement therapies (creams, pellets, pills, patches) and consult your medical oncologist about what is safe and what is certainly not. Remember, we don't want to feed this cancer and give it wings!

In case you already went through menopause (the hot flashes, the crabbiness), well, you may just be welcoming menopause round two.

Also, there is a good chance you are thinking, Estrogen receptor? No problem. I have no ovaries. Or I went through menopause like four decades ago, and now I grow a beard if I don't wax. Sorry gals, you can't skip this section. Our bodies make estrogen outside of the ovaries in multiple tissues. One of the offenders? Those cute little love handles you've been meaning to off-load. That's right. Adipose tissue (colloquially known as fat) makes estrogen in men and women. Bummer, right? Tune in though. It's a smaller amount of estrogen, but it sure is important to your hormone receptor-positive breast cancer.

Let's focus on the positive first. Blocking the signal to those estrogen receptors is like starving the cancer of food (die little beasty!). It has been shown to decrease local-regional recurrence (which is cancer coming back in your breast/armpit nodes), and it has been shown to increase survival. (Hooray! Big shout-out to the scientists that discovered these drugs.) Remember, with any medication out there, we all experience its effects differently. Also remember that with any drug out there, we all experience its effects differently! No, that's not a typo. I need you to pull up a chair and listen! There are some people who become violently ill from Acetaminophen. Some people skate through chemo, go to the gym every day, and work full time. WE ARE ALL DIFFERENT. So please do not listen to your online blog about how anti-estrogen drugs made life a living hell! While that may be true for some; it's not true for all. So give it a try and see how it affects you before you pass judgment. For some women it's like taking a multivitamin. Unfortunately, this boring lack of response does not empower women to shout, "Tamoxifen affects me zero" all over the internet.

All right. Kicking the soapbox to the side, let's move on.

For the premenopausal ladies out there, the first drug of choice is Tamoxifen (and sometimes aromatase inhibitors used in combination with ovarian suppression).

For the post-menopausal ladies out there, the primary drug of choice is aromatase inhibitors (there are several) and sometimes Tamoxifen.

Tamoxifen

Do not take this drug when pregnant, trying to get pregnant, or while breastfeeding. Studies on this wonder drug started in the 1970s; it was approved for cancer treatment in 1980 and later for prevention in 1998. Since then, millions of women (and some men) have taken it. You may be thinking this "wonder drug" is a bit of an oversell if it's going to make you go through early menopause or a second menopause. But consider this: it reduces the risk of your cancer returning or new cancer forming by up to 50 percent. Thank you! What else can it do? you may wonder? Well, it can shrink your cancer, or it can slow or stop the growth of metastatic disease (cancer that has left the breast). While we are on a positive roll, it can also prevent bone loss after menopause and lower cholesterol.

You'll notice there is a long list of medications that do not play nice in the sandbox with tamoxifen. Your doctor will need to make sure the medicines you are on are compatible.

The main side effect of tamoxifen is menopausal symptoms. (If you are one of those ladies that get the "who put me in an oven" hot flashes, take some comfort in knowing that women with hot flashes are less likely to have their cancer come back. Go get some ice packs, fans, and then get naked—in private.) After you gather your fighting tools, march on!

Rare Side effects of Tamoxifen:

- Blood clots: this risk is on par with the risk of blood clots from oral contraceptive pills.

- Uterine cancer: itty bitty risk (like real small) and way smaller than the risk of your breast cancer coming back if you don't take it! Remember, risks and benefits, risks and benefits. You're likely thinking, "Kick that saying to the curb already. Let's talk risk-free benefits!" Sorry, sister, there's always a price to pay for anything in life.

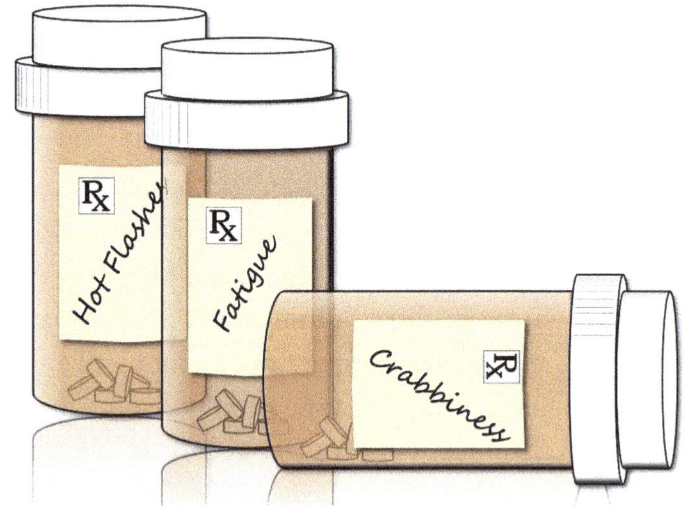

Here's an interesting side note on tamoxifen: some high-risk women without breast cancer take it to try to prevent ever getting cancer!

Aromatase Inhibitors

Arimidex, Aromasin, Femara

These are superior to tamoxifen in clinical trials and are therefore the preferred medication. In case some of you premenopausal nosy pants are perusing this section and wondering, Why isn't this for me? Well, these medications are no match for your ovary estrogen factories. Because of this, they are generally only for the postmenopausal ladies with a critical asterisk . . . ovarian suppression. Premenopausal women can suppress their ovaries with medication and then take aromatase inhibitors. Conversely, if you go through menopause while taking tamoxifen, sound the trumpets and make the switch. Also, don't get pregnant or breastfeed on these puppies; they are no good for embryos.

The main side effects of aromatase inhibitors:

These overall have fewer side effects than tamoxifen (no blood clots, stroke, or endometrial cancer). Still, no medication is without a catch, you postmenopausal marvels! The significant side effect here is osteoporosis. (Alert: It's time for a DEXA scan. This checks for bone density to detect osteopenia or osteoporosis—also known as weakening of the bones.) The other main side effect? Joint pain.

All right, ladies, let's get real for a moment. So, you tried one of these meds and you hate it. You simply cannot live like this. You won't live like this. I hear you! Long life is important, but the quality of life is equally as important, if not more so. I gotcha, so talk to your medical oncologist. They may be able to recommend a reduced dose or switch you to another medication. Don't give up yet. And don't quietly toss the pills into the fire (that you cannot stand close to because you are sweating again and crying and eating ice cream). You have options. Phone a friend . . . may I recommend your medical oncologist?

Fertility

If you have plans for motherhood on the horizon, call in the experts. You should certainly talk with someone who knows their way around retrieving, freezing, and banking eggs; this is no small feat. There are many factors to consider, from out-of-pocket costs (yep!) to egg retrieval timing (and the possible delay in cancer treatments). Additionally, pregnancy is not recommended while on anti-HER2 therapy (which is recommended for a full year) or anti-estrogen therapy (recommended for five to ten years). While conceiving and carrying a child may seem impossible after the last sentence, remember that women do have babies after breast cancer. Read it again: women do have babies after breast cancer. Gather up all the information so that you can start making the decisions that are right for you.

Oncotype Dx Breast Recurrence Score ®

This section is for those ladies with early-stage hormone receptor-positive and HER2 negative cancer. Period! If you are ER and PR negative and/or HER2 positive . . . move on!

There are several tests available to determine the tenacity of this little beastie cancer. And there will be more that come on the market. One of the most widely used is the Oncotype Dx Breast Recurrence score ®.

Chemotherapy in this group of women was once based on the primary tumor's size, whether the cancer skipped town and went to the lymph nodes, the grade, etc. Now, thankfully, we have a much better way to gauge who gets chemo because the intention is always to treat those who benefit the most and spare those who won't benefit any unwanted side-effects. This fantastic test tells you if you will benefit from chemotherapy.

Ta-da! It even gives you the percentage of benefit—for *you*!

To qualify for this test, you need to fit some criteria. You need to be a candidate for chemo (based on your overall health and age). You need to have early-stage hormone-positive and HER2 negative cancer, along with some other factors that your medical oncologist will take into account. If your medical oncologist decides that this is the test for you, then a piece of your cancer (that is sitting in the pathology lab in a bucket) is sent off to a lab to look at the cancer's genetics. Hold on a minute! You are looking at the recipe (DNA) for the cancer cookies (cells)? Yes! And this is not the same as the genetic testing for the BRCA genes (that test looks at the genes you were born with—your original wonderful woman recipe).

The Oncotype Dx ® lab looks at the recipe that went awry, the cancer cell recipe. They test the cancer cells for twenty-one genes; five of those genes are quality control genes, and sixteen genes are the ones being tested. These are resulted as a number score. That number score places you in a high (girl, you need some chemo), intermediate (eh, you may need some chemo depending on your age), or low category (Celebrate! No chemo for you!).

If your score comes back in the low group, there is no survival advantage from chemotherapy. Get on your estrogen blocker and don't look back (and stay on that estrogen blocker). If your score comes back high, chemotherapy will improve your survival. Curse the side effects; be thankful for the benefits and proceed to the infusion room, sister!

If you are intermediate, then it gets a little more complicated and depends on your age. For those under fifty, chemotherapy may be recommended, especially if you are on the high side of intermediate. (If you are over fifty, no chemo! Yay!)

Chemotherapy

Shaken, Not Stirred!

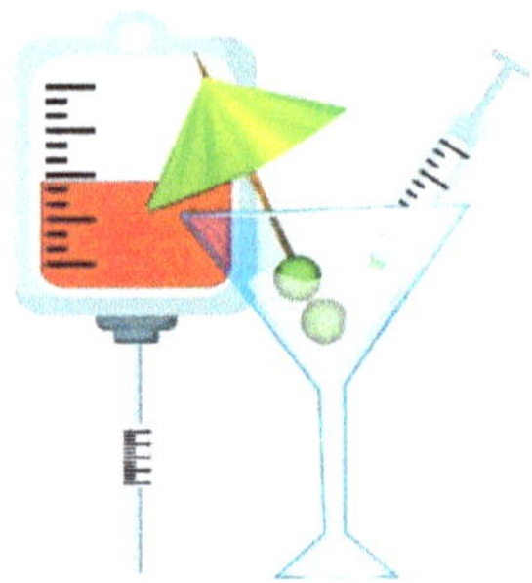

Not everyone needs chemo, so unless your doc recommended chemo, there is no need to waste precious life reading this chapter. Take a deep breath and send some positive vibes to your cancer sisters out there, then you can skip this chapter.

And for you chemo queens, no one wants chemo—no one! But sometimes you need to sharpen the tools you have and get to it! These meds have a bad rap, and there's a good reason. They aren't without some pretty crappy side effects. Some of them can be serious—or rarely, even deadly. But if chemo saves far more lives than it hurts (risk and benefits again—blah, blah), then let's do it.

Most chemotherapy drugs are given just downright weird names. Hard to pronounce, harder to remember; therefore we abbreviate them. And again, this isn't exhaustive. If you are someone with significant medical conditions, or you already have a personal history of taking chemotherapy, you may take the road less traveled. And that's okay! If your recommended combo isn't here, don't fear. This list is not exhaustive of the options available.

ACTHP, ACT, TC, TCHP, and TH is each a chemotherapy recipe, and the letters stand for a chemotherapy or HER2 targeted therapy (which is not technically chemotherapy).

Let's dive in!

Standard Chemotherapy for Breast Cancer

They all kill cancer. Yay for that! They mostly work by damaging the recipe (DNA) to make cookies (cells). Still, I rather like the idea that they are some wayward cookie monster with a penchant for the bad cookies (cancer). Unfortunately, they eat some of the good cookies too, resulting in a-la side effects like hair loss.

There is, of course, a long list of side effects (just like the store-bought pain reliever package insert), but of course, these are a bit more serious. As with all side effects, each person experiences them in differing severity. You usually don't experience *all* the side effects. This section is meant to be read in an "end of new medication commercial" voice:

> "May cause problems with your blood cells (impaired immune cells and increased risk of bleeding issues), GI issues (nausea, vomiting, poor appetite, mouth sores), and hair and nail problems."

What on earth does this all mean? Am I going to be laid up in bed, bald, vomiting, and bleeding? (I know I sound a bit harsh, but it's what some of you are thinking!) The short answer is yes, there will be some rough days, but not all will be bad, and even the bad days might not be as bad as you may be imagining. There are cool caps for hair (but your hair still won't be the same). There are excellent meds for nausea (thank you, science!), and your doc will be drawing your blood to check labs before you get each dose of chemo to make sure your immune system and blood clotting ability are ready for the next dose. If your lab numbers dip too low, you may be confronted with a couple of different scenarios. You may be asked to go home and come back in a week. You may get some extra meds. And you may get an infection that could be mild, or that could land you in the hospital. Take things as they come. The majority of women complete their planned chemotherapy. Be patient with your body. Oh, and if you still have periods, expect the chemo to make these irregular or stop altogether.

These guys are almost uniformly given via IV; therefore long-term IV access may be necessary. This usually comes in the form of a "port" (see the section on ports on page 126).

Now, a final warning before you proceed. Have you ever started to itch after someone mentioned lice or told a story about a spider crawling on them? Well, the brain is powerful, and you may not want to be focusing too much on the side effects. I urge you to proceed with caution.

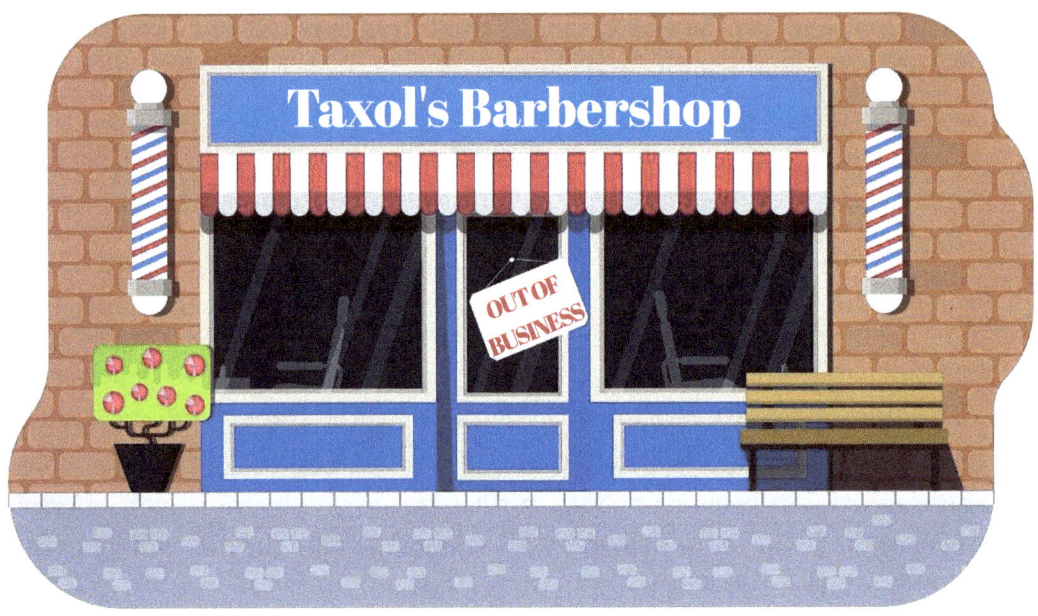

"Am I going to lose my hair?"

There are certainly some strategies to minimize hair loss, but the general rule is, yes. Some of you will look downright cute bald! Regardless, you have options. You can spend some serious dough and get a wig that looks close to whatever your regular do is. Or you can step outside your comfort zone and go bold (think pink bob or leopard headscarf). You can also go Q-ball bald (but please wear sunscreen outside), or just pick a comfy hat. Whatever you chose, realize that it's temporary (although a small group of women do have permanent hair thinning).

A. Adriamycin (given IV)

It's a cancer killer! That's excellent news, but unfortunately, like a bad boyfriend, it can also break your heart. Therefore, like a good bartender/ therapist, your medical oncologist will be doing deep dives, checking in with your heart. This will happen with that trusty ultrasound again. (Score #2 for ultrasounds!)

C. Cytoxan (oral or IV) or Carboplatin (IV)

Cytoxan is usually given in combination with other chemotherapies (and shares the usual suspects of side effects).

Carboplatin is notorious for nerve damage or neuropathy. This typically affects fingertips and toes. Sometimes this is permanent, and sometimes you recover partially or entirely. Kidney damage is also another side effect.

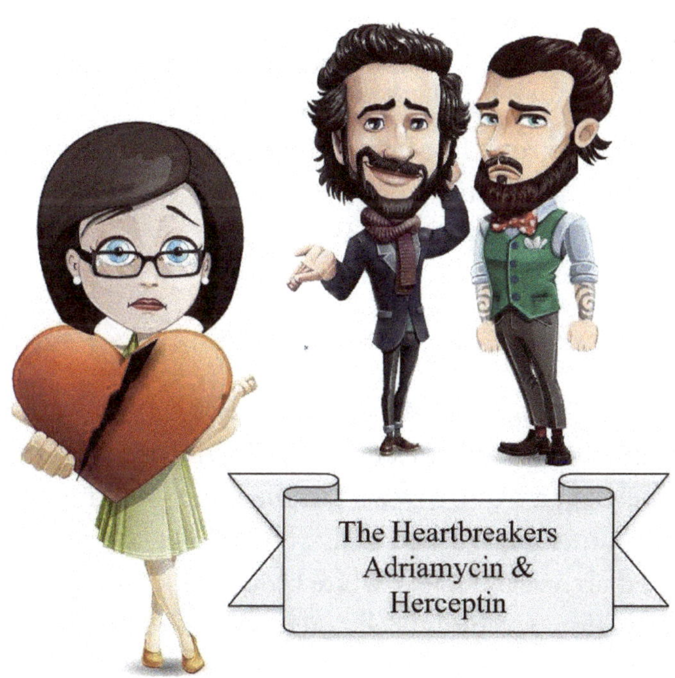

T. Taxol or Taxotere (both are given IV)

Both are given with "solvents" or extra medications to break down these drugs so that they can enter the bloodstream. These solvents can cause their own side effects and can make these hard to tolerate and cause reactions.

Taxol is usually given in combination with something else. Again, it's associated with the standard list of fun side effects, and then it layers on some more. This guy may give you neuropathy (neuro- what?): damage to nerves. This typically affects fingertips and toes. Sometimes this is permanent, and sometimes you recover partially or completely.

Taxotere also causes neuropathy (see above) as well as fluid retention, fatigue (I know—you may be thinking—too freakin' late. I am fatigued and haven't even started!), bone/joint/muscle pain, watery eyes. Oh, and these guys are responsible for hairloss too. . .

HER2 targeted Therapy

If you are HER2-neu negative, move along. There's nothing to see here, Ms. Nosy!

All right, these medications are like attack drones specifically made to target those HER2 satellite dishes. Kachaw! Thank you, smart scientists! HER2 positive cancers are bad business; they like to grow. But before your heart skips another beat, we have a way to exploit that: Bing. Bang. Boom. Poof!

H-Herceptin (IV)

Cancer killer . . . yay! He is going to be around for a year or maybe more. This guy is another potential heartbreaker, which means you are not done with that ultrasound machine yet. You'll likely get a front-row seat to the inner workings of your heart via a painless and quick ultrasound (called an ECHO). Like chemotherapy, you have another reason to have diarrhea and a low white blood cell count (immune cell). You may also develop anemia (low red blood cell count, these are the oxygen carriers) and abdominal pain.

P-Perjeta (IV)

Cancer killer . . . yay again! This drug is typically given together with Herceptin. No getting pregnant, sister! Much the same as the others—at this point, I think you get the message. Diarrhea, hair loss, low white blood cell count, nausea, fatigue, rash, and neuropathy. Nothing new to see here.

Ports . . . ports everywhere, but not a sailboat or wine spritzer in sight!

For those of you ladies signing up for the big-guns chemo or the long haul with anti-HER2 treatment, your doc will likely recommend that you have a port placed. This is a device to provide you with long-term IV access to receive your chemotherapy without burning up and poking the veins in your arms. It is usually placed by your surgeon or an interventional radiologist on the day of your first chemo or several days to weeks before your first chemotherapy. But what the heck is it?

It's basically a small reservoir under the skin (the size of a water bottle cap) with a small tube that runs under the skin from this reservoir to a vein (a little smaller than IV tubing). It goes into the vein and down toward the heart. The tip of the tubing sits right outside the heart in the largest vein in your body (the vena cava). When you have your treatment, the nurse places a needle into the reservoir to administer the chemotherapy. That noxious, albeit life-saving chemo then goes into the reservoir, through the tubing, and out into the bloodstream at a place where the chemotherapy can be quickly diluted (so as not to injure the small veins). At the completion of its use, it can be removed. Wham, bam, thank you, ma'am.

Support Medications

These guys are here to help squash the adverse effects of chemotherapy so that you don't feel so darn miserable. Some of these meds help your immune system rebound from the chemotherapy quicker! These little gems have dramatically changed how people experience chemo. You've got your anti-emetics (the nausea squashers): Zofran, Phenergan, Reglan, Compazine, as well as a few others. You've got your white blood cell mobilizers: Neulasta and Neupogen type stuff. These guys help your immune system mobilize from the bone marrow (where they are made) and into circulation, where they can do their job. You've got Benadryl (yes, the stuff you can get over the counter can work wonders) and steroids (these babies can make you feel pretty darn good). I am telling you, chemo is a lot more tolerable nowadays.

Which one comes first? Surgery or chemotherapy?

Bottom line: survival is the same. It doesn't matter who goes first (with some exceptions).

For some, it's a little bit of a "chicken or egg" thing. Each case is different, and your surgeon and medical oncologist need to chat. Does your medical oncologist need information from the surgery (like, "How big is this thing really?" and "Are there lymph nodes involved?") to help them decide if you need chemo, or what concoction of chemotherapy you need. Or does the surgeon need chemo to shrink the cancer to make surgery feasible and decrease the chance of positive margins (think inflammatory breast cancer, large cancers, or cancers trying to cozy up to the chest wall or skin)?

This is a very tricky decision, so leave this one to the experts. If your doc says chemo first and you respond with, "Are you freaking kidding me? I want you to cut this thing out! I don't want to have this cancer in my breast for the next several months!" Hold on. Take a breath and turn on your listening ears. (I know you mommies have said this before.) There are some really good reasons to do chemo first.

1. Is this chemo working? Well, if your cancer is sitting in a bucket in a lab, ain't nobody going to know how well the chemotherapy is working on it. Conversely, if it's sitting in your breast, we can see how it responds to the chemo. Is it shrinking? Is it growing? If it's growing, we jump off the chemo ship and board the surgery steam liner or change tack on the type of chemo. When you finish chemo and we take that sucker out, we can really see how well the chemo worked. Some women have "complete pathologic responses." Decoded, that means "No cancer left! The chemo melted that cancer away. We can all breathe a little better knowing that this group of women has a better prognosis." If you don't have this response, fear not; we still gained valuable information. Ta-da! If you had a partial response, we know that you may benefit from more chemo (and that can mean living longer). (Well, shucka-dillies, that is not what you wanted to hear.) But the silver lining is now you know that you will benefit from more chemo. (If you'd had surgery first, you would have missed this opportunity for more chemo. I know . . . sad face.)

2. Answer me this: What's more important? Your whole body or your breast? Well, if you are scratching your head, let me lay it out. If you had to choose one, which one would you choose to live without? Breast or body? (I know I'm a bit sassy, but this is a huge point!) Okay, so chemo treats the whole body (including the breast), and surgery only treats your breast. Do you want chemo or surgery first now? (Hint: you can live without a breast; you cannot live without your body.)

Got it! Chemo first, full steam ahead. Woah, not so fast, friend. There are some really good reasons for surgery first:

The information gained by surgical pathology can change the whole chemo plan. Imaging does give us an idea of size, but for those of you who have seen your mammogram, ultrasound, and breast MRI breast cancer size estimations, you know that these don't quite line up . . . and neither will your pathology. And ladies, size matters. Size expectations go both ways—small on imaging and large on pathology (it's not the norm, but a mass that is 1 cm on imaging can become 4 cm or more on pathology) or, conversely, a cancer can be large on imaging and small on pathology (4 cm on imaging becomes 1 cm or less on pathology). Are you thinking this sounds like a raw deal? You're telling me we are flying blind with some dirty, rotten lying imaging? Well, first you need to remember that this is not the norm; it is the exception when that happens. We make our decisions with the information that we have at the moment. That's the best we can do until time travel is invented. Second, lymph nodes. Lymph nodes can look normal on imaging, but they can certainly have cancer in them. We don't know unless a sentinel lymph node biopsy is performed. For a lymph node to look abnormal on imaging, the cancer in them needs to be big enough to change the size or shape of the lymph node.

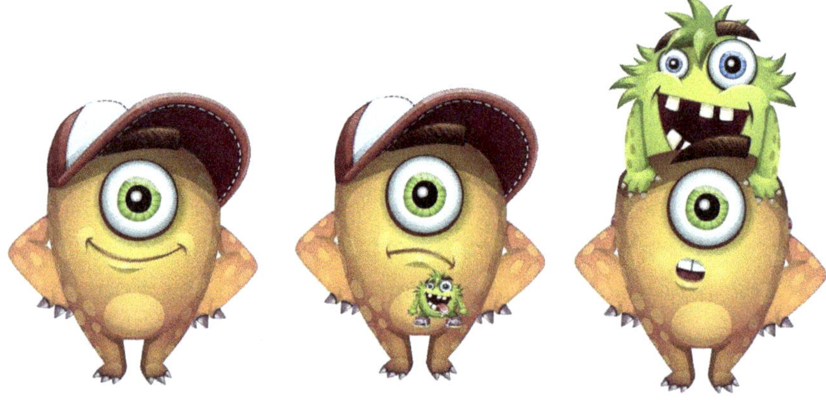

Normal Lymph Node Normal Shape and Size

Little bit of Cancer: Normal Shape and Size

Big amount of Cancer: Abnormal shape and/or size

Are you thinking, You've sold me on both. Chemo first or surgery first—or maybe not? Well, that is why it's a decision to be made with the help of your A-Team. They will present you with their recommendation and then, of course, it's your body, girlfriend. Listen, meditate, pray, etc. But please don't ask Dr. Google. He hasn't read your chart, and as you now know, there are reasons for both. There will be stories on both sides.

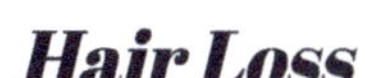

Hair Loss

"Is there some way to prevent hair loss? Neuropathy? How do I get through this chemo unscathed?" Well, there are certainly tools to help with these, but it's not a perfect system.

"Cold caps," otherwise known as scalp hypothermia (or brrrrrrr! cold, cold, cold head).

This is an FDA-approved device that has been used in the US since 2015 (and in Europe for several decades). How does it work? Cold constricts blood flow. The goal is to minimize the blood flow to the scalp during chemotherapy (so that the chemo in your bloodstream doesn't end up spending so much time around those precious but temperamental hair follicles). The idea has been around since the 1970s, when people started using ice packs. But before you go running off in search of this therapy, please recognize that it is far from perfect. Also, take note that it's expensive and not always covered by insurance.

This same idea can be applied to hands and toes to prevent neuropathy (nerve damage).

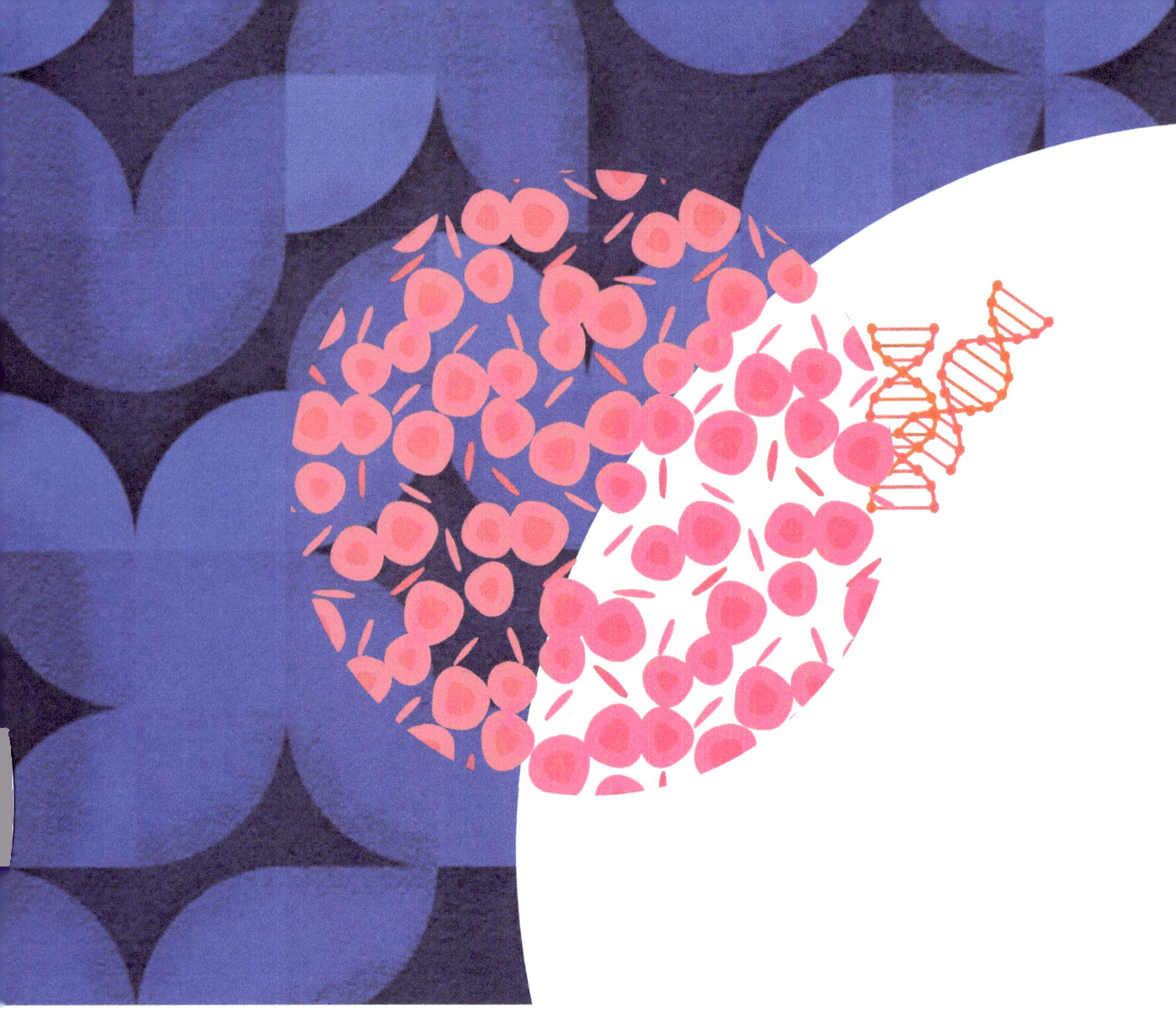

SCIENCE SIMPLIFIED!

You might be thinking, How does this poison work? Well, in the simplest form of understanding, it kills fast-dividing cells. Fast-dividing cells mean cancer, but this also means the normally fast-dividing cells of the body are at risk—your gut cells and hair follicles. But how? Remember that cookie recipe (DNA) that gets copied every time you make more cookies (make more cells)? Chemotherapy basically disrupts this process; it's like having a pen without ink. No ink, no recipe, no new cookies.

Some chemotherapies insert a couple of extra letters in every word until the recipe just doesn't make sense. This doesn't matter as much for a long-lived cell (say, brain cells that may last your whole life). But for colon cells that recycle every four days, that chemotherapy will cause some trouble (enter side effects).

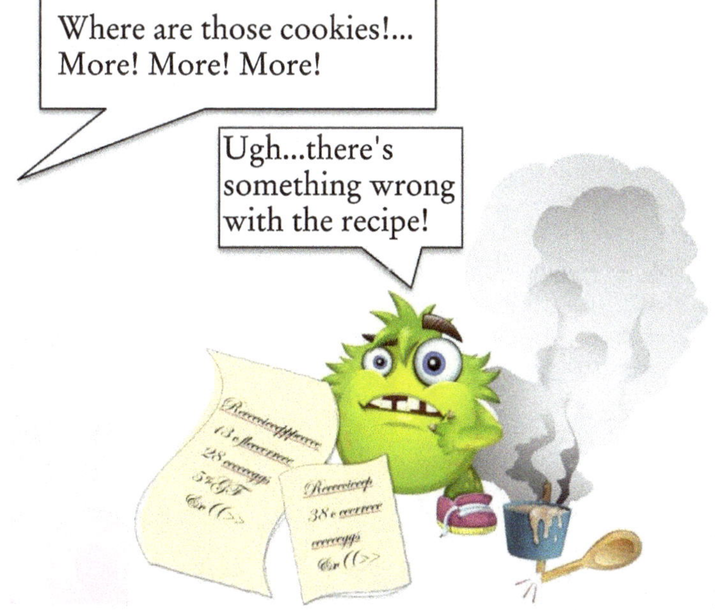

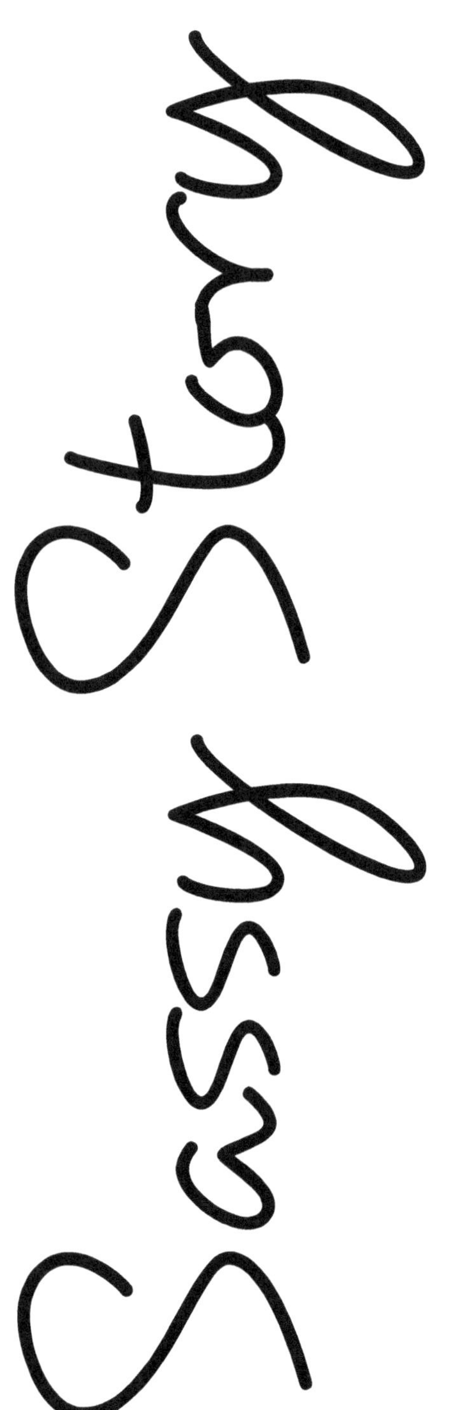

Who Invented This Poison?

The first chemotherapy agent arrived on the market in 1958. For something that is so widely used today, it's pretty hard to imagine that it wasn't around sixty-five years ago. Interestingly, that very first chemo drug is still widely used today!

The specific agents to target receptors came considerably later. Tamoxifen (the anti-estrogen pill) didn't have her coming-out party until the 1980s. Herceptin (anti-HER2 receptor therapy) became available in 1998, and Perjeta (anti-HER2 receptor therapy) is really still the new kid on the block (2017).

As for those magic meds that helped you survive the chemo? Phenergan is an oldie but goodie, first invented in the 1940s and FDA approved in 1951. Reglan was FDA approved in 1979. Zofran was developed in England in the 1980s and approved by the FDA in 1991. Compazine was FDA approved in 1999.

FAQs:

Frequently Asked Questions

Q. Am I really going to lose my hair?

A. Pretty much, yeah. At the very least, it's likely to thin even with the best prevention.

Q. Am I going to vomit all the time?

A. Likely not; there are some great meds to prevent this!

Q. Will I just feel like crap all the time?

A. Usually, days two to four after chemo are the "worst." Remember, everyone is different, and some women work full time throughout their chemo treatments.

Q. Can I go to work?

A. Yes! Listen to your body. There are plenty of women that, either by choice or necessity, continue to work!

Q. Can I have sex?

A. Yes (for the most part)! Cancer is not sexually transmitted, and chemo is generally not sexually transmitted. But please remember that you have enough on your plate! Talk to your doc about contraception options!

The BIG day! A lot of sitting . . .

1. You have your port, or your doc says a peripheral IV (arm) is enough for your cocktail. You have been prescribed the support meds, and you have them in hand. You have been given some other instructions like what to eat, what not to eat, what supplements you should or shouldn't take, and what precautions you will need to take in the days following chemo.

2. Your doc may ask you to take meds before chemo or place numbing cream over your port (which is then covered with a dressing). Take them.

3. You will need a driver for at least the first time or two until you know how *you* handle the chemo.

4. You show-up and check-in . . . for the first time. Like the first day of a new job, what is now foreign will become your commonplace. You will sign some forms consenting to the risks of chemotherapy.

5. You will have blood drawn (or maybe you already had blood drawn) to check your labs and make sure you are in your prime for chemo. You will have your blood pressure, heart rate, and weight recorded.

6. You will be shown to an infusion room with comfy chairs, IV poles, snacks, and hopefully a view.

7. Here comes the IV, or your port will be accessed (a needle goes through the skin and into the port). You may be given

some support meds through the IV. Then, if you are a cold cap girl, here comes the brain freeze and may some cold mittens too.

8. The chemo starts, and you wait . . . usually for a couple of hours while the chemo goes into your body (pew, pew!). Goodbye cancer.

9. You may feel nothing; you may feel awful. It's one of those wait-and-see moments. Some people read, watch tv, chat with friends, work, sleep, etc. Nurses will be checking on you and checking your vitals.

10. When you are done, the IV is removed, or the port is de-accessed. You may be asked to hang out for a little while to make sure you feel okay.

11. You go home, take some more support meds. Those meds may include the meds to boost your immune cells.

12. Days two through four may be rough, but you have those meds to help you deal with symptoms. Take them! Then you slowly feel better until the next one. Rinse and repeat.

Let's Review

- You will get an individualized treatment plan! It's not *all* about how to treat the cancer (the size, receptors, and lymph node status). It's about you and your body too. All the risks and benefits will be weighed before a treatment plan is finalized.

- Not everyone with breast cancer needs chemotherapy.

- Not everyone with breast cancer gets the same chemotherapy.

- Sometimes chemotherapy comes before surgery.

- Chemotherapy saves far more lives than it hurts!

- You are going to lose some or all of your hair.

- You may feel like you are going through menopause (either for the first or second time).

- You may need a port for chemotherapy administration (but not always).

Short-term and long-term side effects are way more manageable than in the past! There are a lot of tricks to try for hot flashes, neuropathy, and vaginal dryness (yes, I said it). The only way to begin to fix those pesky side effects is to talk to your medical oncologist.

Thoughts and Questions About Chemo, The Pill, and HER2 Therapy

Words from Your Sisters:

You are not alone!

By now, the doctor visits were the "social" part of my calendar. I even had girls at work give me Marti Gras beads since I was whipping my shirt up so much!

Survivor Sister

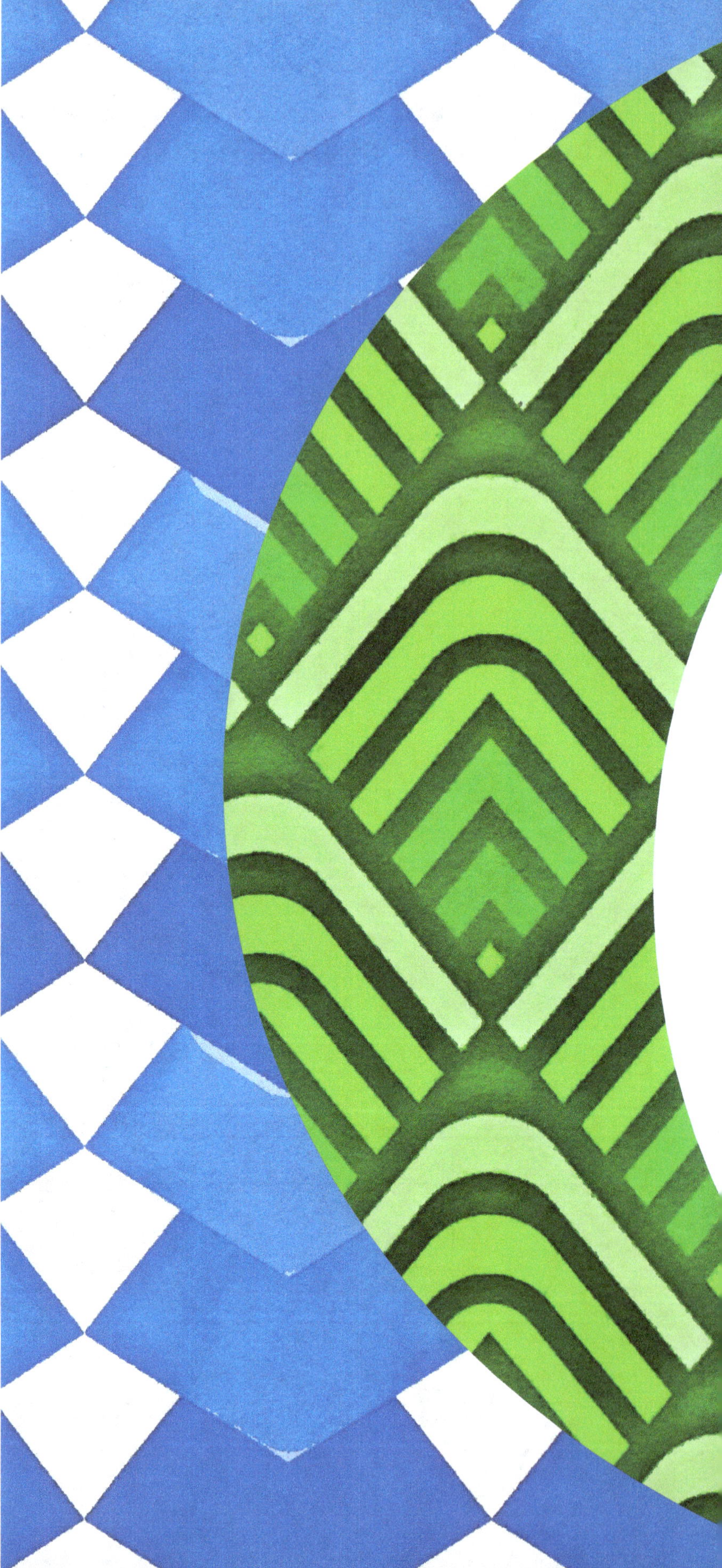

Special Cases

What About Me?

Well, having cancer sucks! Sometimes it seems to happen at one of those moments in life where the refried beans are quite literally hitting the fan on multiple fronts. You may feel like a beleaguered, battle-tested soldier who isn't quite sure yet how or when or where the war will end. Again, remember that you are not the first pregnant lady, a young mama with young kids, a caregiver for a family member with special needs, or a gal with a messy, abusive divorce. Life is not always a warm slice of pie with melted vanilla ice cream on top. (I know you don't need me to tell you this!) Sometimes it's a hot flaming mess on your front doorstep. In this instance, no amount of tender- loving prose is going to snap you back to "good." Sometimes only the passage of time, or learning to gently and lovingly embrace a love for yourself, or . . . well, crap. Help me fill in the blank here! This section is for you, ladies—a little pep talk of sorts. It sure isn't going to solve your problems, but it will give you some info and maybe, just maybe give you a push in the right direction.

I'm Pregnant

Help!

You are not alone. You are not alone. You are not alone. You have the same survival rate as your nonpregnant counterparts! Yay for this! And every year, healthy babies are born after their mommies undergo chemotherapy and surgery. You can keep that baby healthy and carry him or her to term, mama! You can do this. Of course, there are some very specific, just-for-mama care decisions that your A-team will need to make, and they largely depend on where you are in your pregnancy. The bottom line is that chemotherapy can be given after the first trimester. Surgery can be done in any trimester. Radiation cannot be done at any time during pregnancy. And sentinel lymph node biopsy has some limitations in pregnancy. (Remember the blue dye? Well, it's not for you, mama.) You need a coordinated care team. But, you can do this!

Inflammatory Breast Cancer

My Breast Is Red!

Did you wake up one day and some or all of your breast was red? Maybe you thought it was an infection or rash at first, but the redness didn't go away with antibiotics. If you had to pick a flavor of breast cancer, this would not be your first choice, but, as with any diagnosis, it's the first step to laying out a path to a cure. In this case, the path is clearly laid out. There is very little deviation from this treatment regiment. You are looking at chemotherapy for several months. Three to four weeks to recover from chemo. Then surgery is a modified radical mastectomy. (This means goodbye to the breast and the lymph nodes under the arm.) After another three to four weeks of healing from surgery, you get radiation. And then (...you are thinking, "No and then!") the anti-estrogen pill or anti-HER2 therapy, depending on your receptors. Period. There's the plan! Go forward, don't look back, and conquer!

Paget's Disease

My Nipple Looks Weird!

Did you notice that one of your nipples just does not look the same? Well, this is breast cancer that has spilled out of the duct and onto the skin of the nipple. It is commonly, but not always associated with breast cancer in the underlying ducts near the nipple. So, it's essential to rule out cancer inside the breast too.

Phyllodes

Listen doc, I was told I have breast cancer, but you haven't mentioned the one I have yet! Well, the origins of this odd word are also Greek, meaning "leaf-like." Have you ever seen a split-leaf philodendron? Phyllodes comes in three flavors: benign, borderline, and malignant. Most of these are benign, but you aren't here because you have a benign phyllodes. Malignant Phyllodes are *rare* and they get their own rule book! When it comes to surgery, your options are largely the same- but we typically aim for wider margins and leave the lymph nodes alone (these suckers hop into the blood stream before they go looking for lymphatic channels). Radiation and chemo are still on the table but, again, the rule book for when these are considered will be different. Call in the A-Team and listen-up for your individualized plan!

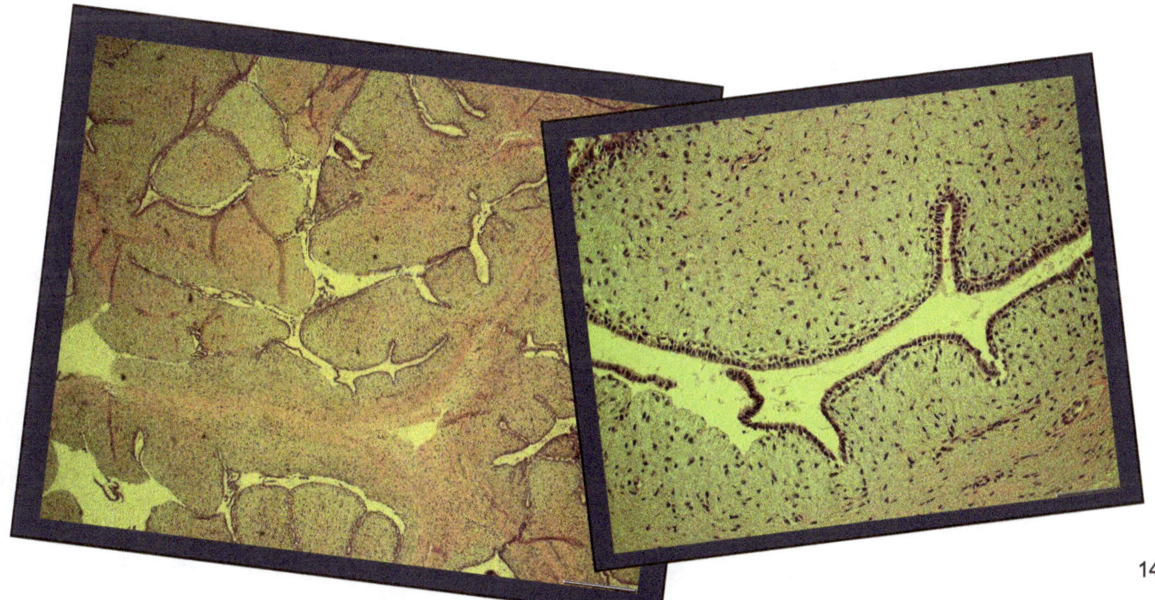

Words from Your Sisters:

You are not alone!

I hear some women say that breast cancer was the best thing to happen to them. I don't agree with that. It is awful and devastating. It may come back, and you may die from it. It's the first time I have been faced with a possible death sentence. To get through this journey, I was busy with positive goals. I had a lot of people send me wonderful presents, cards, and cookies when they found out about my journey. I love people, and that was given back to me! Thanks to all my friends and family!

Survivor Sister

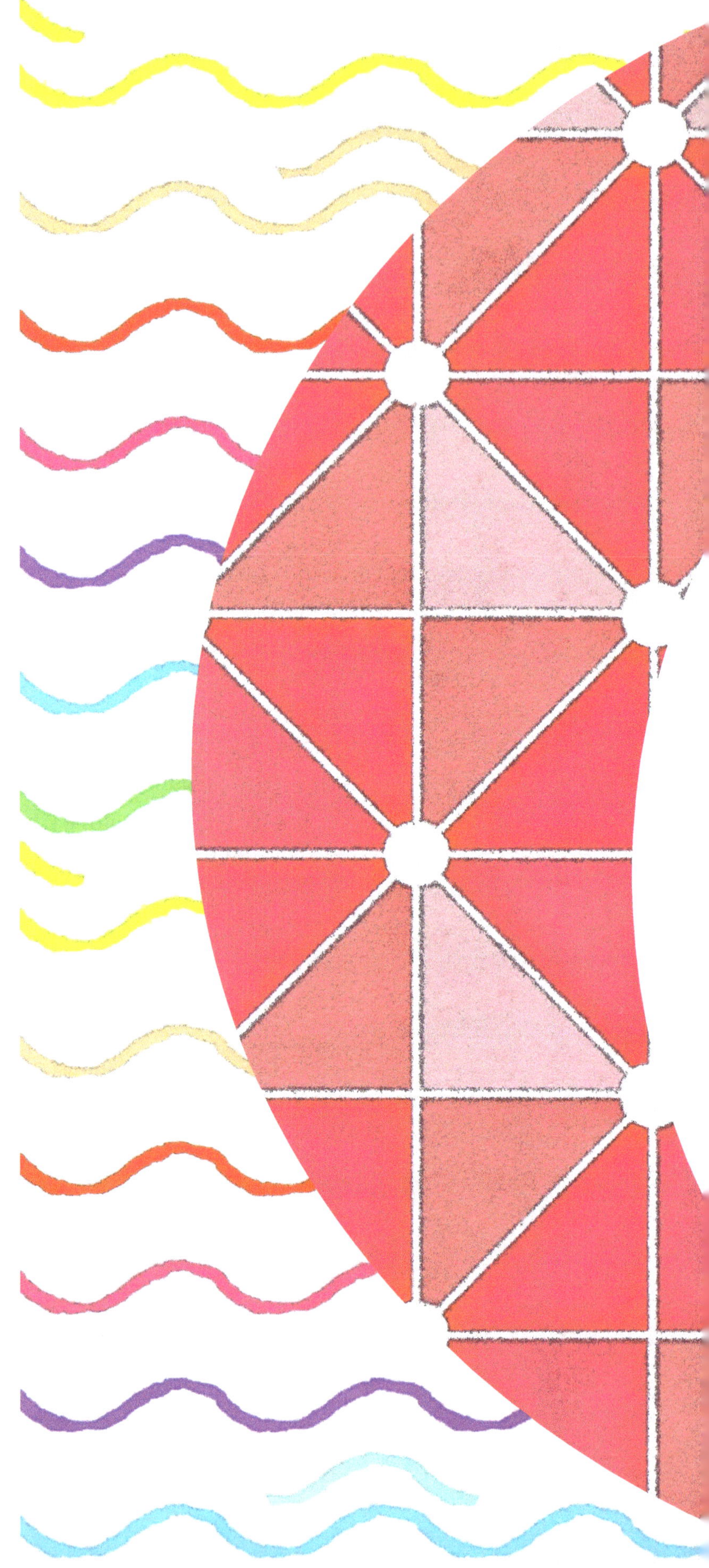

Stage IV

My Cancer Flew the Coop!

Someone told you that your cancer is travel-happy and has spread outside your breast and armpit lymph nodes. All right, breathe. Breathe again! (Warning: if you read this book too fast, you might just hyperventilate with all this coaching to take deep breaths.)

First, your stage IV breast cancer is not the same as the next lady's stage IV breast cancer. Let me repeat that again: your breast cancer is not the same as someone else's breast cancer! Period. If you feel compelled at some point to say, "But my neighbor knows a lady who . . ." Stop! No comparing.

Next, there are no crystal balls here; no doctor will be able to predict the day of your death. We are surprised all the time by the person who defies the odds. And remember, they are just that—odds. They aren't what will happen to you; they are what happens if you look at thousands of women (all of which have different breast cancers with different combinations of receptors and different sites of metastasis).

Stage IV covers the gals with a 5 mm breast tumor and a single small metastatic bone lesion. Stage IV also covers the ladies with a breast entirely replaced with cancer with innumerable bone lesions, liver lesions, and brain lesions. Your outlook will depend on things like who you are and how your tumor responds to therapy. There are certainly women who leave this earth much too quickly after a diagnosis of stage IV breast cancer. However, some women have been living with stage IV breast cancer for over a decade (albeit these are the minority). Where you fit in this whole mess is up to your tumor's biology, which is likely to be entirely unpredictable at the time of diagnosis. What do I mean by *biology of the tumor*? That's medical jargon for how tenacious those cancer cells are. Are they meek wallflowers that will shrivel up the moment they see some treatment (fingers crossed), or are they Roman soldiers with fortified defenses (bah)? You are not going to like this, but only time will tell. I don't have a magic sentence for you to read that will make all your anxieties dissipate, answer all your family members' questions, and stop the flow of tears. Sorry, sister, I cannot promise you that everything will be all right. And if you are downright pissed at this or are wondering how you can still have tears left in your body to cry . . . no one can promise anyone a perfect outcome.

Everyone will deal with this differently. Everyone has different support systems and belief systems; there is no wrong answer to how you will deal with this. Some women may jump ship and fly somewhere tropical. ("The hell with this! I am drinking margaritas by the pool until I run out of time or money!") Some women will start their journeys to flagship cancer hospitals to enroll in the latest drug trial (paying it forward and hoping to garner some benefit in the meantime). The first piece of advice I have for you is to put in the time to talk with all the docs, and consider all the options before you make your decision.

There are people who love you, and it would be a damn shame to rob yourself and them of years with you if you are one of those "lucky" ladies who could have another ten or more years on this earth. Yes, time and quality of life can be two separate things. And yes, your oncologist wants those years to be quality years, not just years (we aren't talking bald and puking). My next piece of advice is to find your entourage or tribe. You're not doing this alone. Even if life feels like a bag of lemons right now and your entourage needs to be your doctors and nurses, you are never as alone as you may feel.

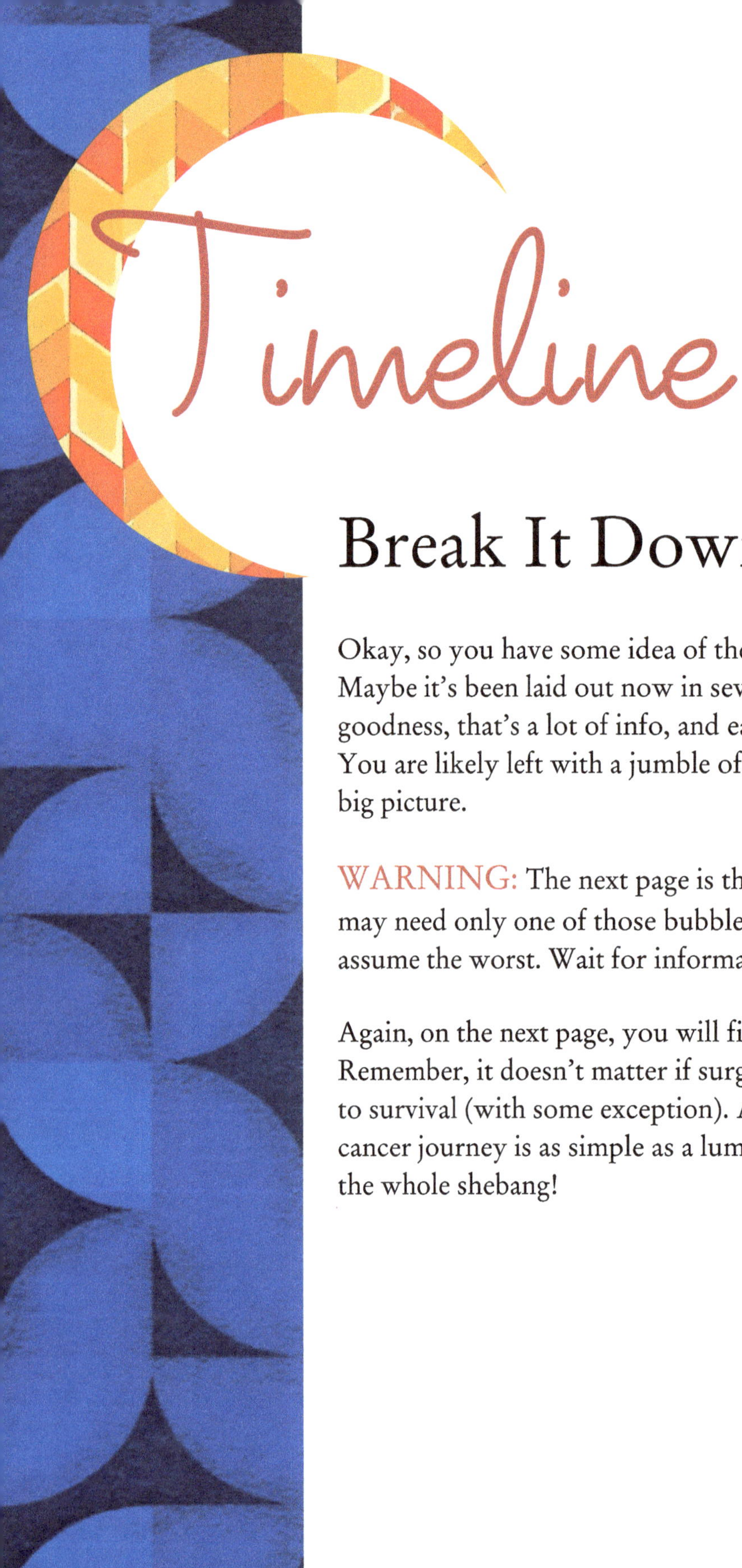

Timeline

Break It Down!

Okay, so you have some idea of the various therapies you need. Maybe it's been laid out now in several doctors' visits. But my goodness, that's a lot of info, and each doc talks about it differently. You are likely left with a jumble of information. Let's talk about the big picture.

WARNING: The next page is the max amount of therapy. You may need only one of those bubbles, so take a deep breath and don't assume the worst. Wait for information from the A-team!

Again, on the next page, you will find the outline for maximal therapy. Remember, it doesn't matter if surgery or chemo is first when it comes to survival (with some exception). Also remember that some women's cancer journey is as simple as a lumpectomy, while some women need the whole shebang!

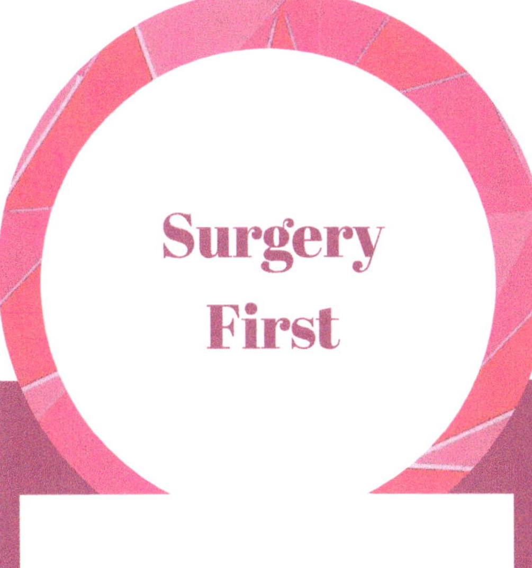

Chemotherapy
First

Surgery

Chemotherapy
2-5 Months

Chemotherapy
2-5 Months

Surgery

Maybe More Chemo

HER2+

HER2 Targeted Therapy
1 year

Radiation
1-7 weeks

ER+ and/or PR+
Estrogen Blocking Pill
5-10 years

Survivorship

My Cancer Care Worksheet

Keeping Track of the Important Things!!!

Type of cancer: (ductal, lobular, mammary, etc)		________________		
Is there more than one cancer?		yes	no	
Grade of cancer 1, 2, or 3:		____________		
Size of cancer:		____________ cm		
Receptors:	Estrogen:	yes	no	
	Progesterone:	yes	no	
	HER2:	yes	no	
Is there cancer in my lymph nodes?		yes	no	maybe
Has it spread to other parts of my body?		yes	no	maybe
Stage of cancer:		____________		
Am I a candidate for lumpectomy?		yes	no	maybe
Am I a candidate for reconstruction?		yes	no	maybe
Do I need chemotherapy?		yes	no	maybe
Should I get chemo first?		yes	no	maybe
Do I need radiation?		yes	no	maybe
Should I get genetic testing?		yes	no	maybe
Will I go home the same day as the surgery?		yes	no	maybe
Do I need a port?		yes	no	maybe

Thoughts and Questions

Words from Your Sisters:

You are not alone!

I called my brother in tears and told him that I just could not do months upon months of chemotherapy. I had completed two rounds and felt like I had been hit by a Mack truck. I just wanted to stop and pretend it all wasn't happening. The words he said kept me going: "You only have to do one more treatment, just one more, after that one you decide if you are doing the next one treatment. Take them one at a time." It helped to break it down into little steps so that I wasn't committing to the marathon at the outset. One step at a time. I made it through all my treatments, one at a time.

Survivor Sister

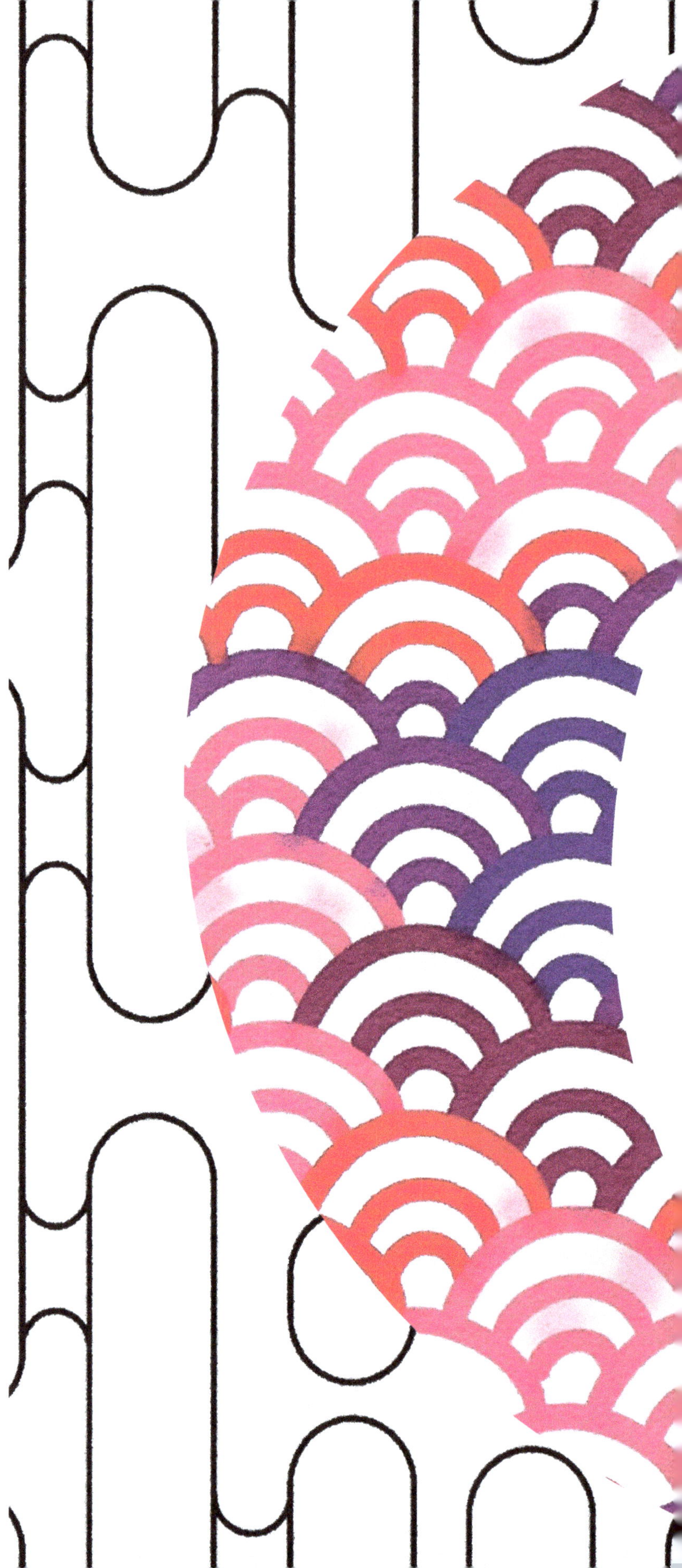

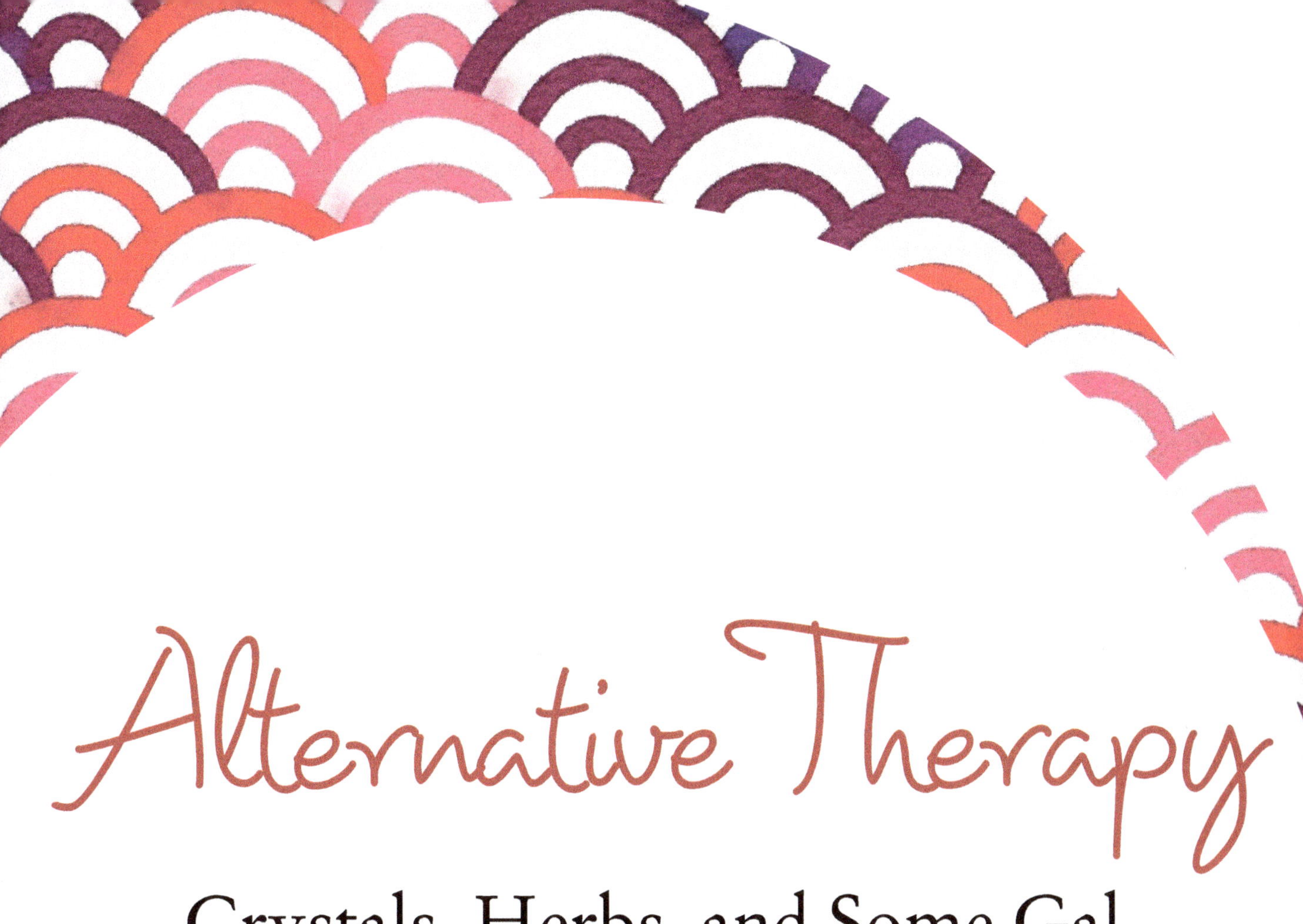

Alternative Therapy

Crystals, Herbs, and Some Gal in Mexico

Alternative therapies are often alluring, but don't let yourself get off track girlfriend. The mind is important, if you want to go on a yoga retreat, smell some incense, and sleep with some crystals, go for it! You need things that help you feel better, feel proactive, and like you are "doing everything that you can." We all know the power of our minds is immense! You might be grasping for control and feeling like you are riding a wild roller coaster you don't remember ever waiting in line for. You have some tough decisions to make. So, sure! Get a massage, mani-pedi, facial, and balance your chakras.

But please, please, please do not substitute crystals or coffee enemas for . . . say . . . chemotherapy. Chemotherapy kills cancer—period. (Yes, it works better for some than others. And yep, there are certainly some downsides.) These other *things* may be touted to cure ugly and make us all look like supermodels while purifying the body of all evil. But come on? If you think that the pharmaceutical companies and doctors fighting cancer wouldn't latch on to something that kills cancer, you are kidding yourself.

Of Course! We can *certainly* cure cancer without side effects!
SNAKE OIL SALESMAN

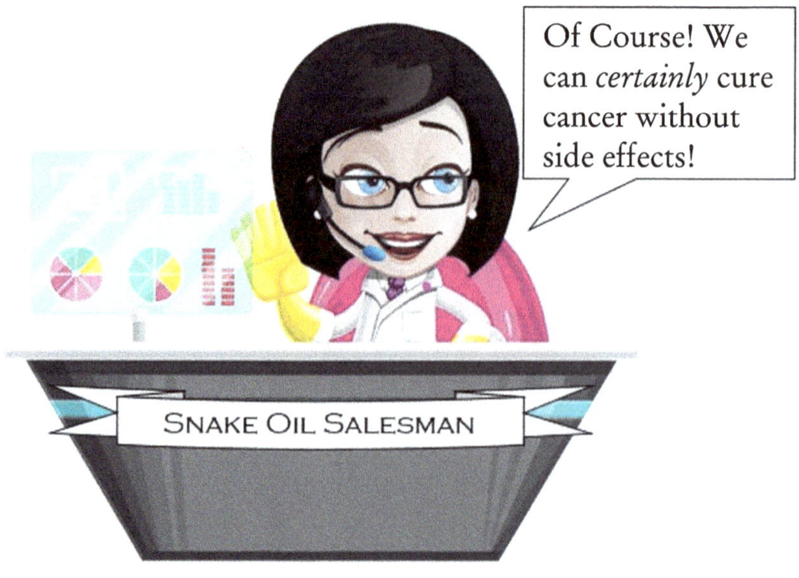

Every cancer doctor has seen too many people (even one person is one too many) go buy snake oil disguised with good intentions and then circle back to "Western" medicine when that fails. Unfortunately, by the time they realize things aren't working is about the time their disease went from curable to . . . well, not curable. Please don't be that person.

Soapbox Moment

Big Pharma spends big bucks developing and selling medications; there is no doubt about it. But if you believe this, then the next logical step is not "they are trying to hide the truth about blueberries!" I beg you to consider the opposite. They are going to get their hands on anything that can help fight cancer, purify it, and dole it out (enter the long list of profitable medications developed from plants). That's exactly how Taxol (aka paclitaxel, a common chemotherapy) eventually came into being.

Now, I am not claiming altruism. But I am asking you to consider that capitalism would drive this gravy train in any direction that works! One in eight women get breast cancer. That's a huge market. No one is going to pass up a chance to develop therapies for this one!

Okay, go do you! It's your body. Be a good steward of that body for yourself and the people that like having you around. Chemo, surgery, and radiation are scary. But girlfriend, if you can make it through these flaming hoops, you'll hopefully be cancer-free and living large again. Do anything short of what is recommended for you, and your chances of living large (cancer-free) may decline. Tough love. Sorry, star princess. But I care about you!

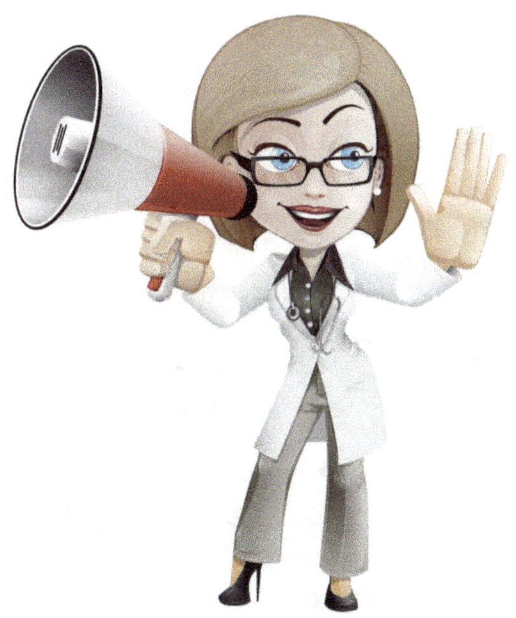

Natural Chemotherapy

Paclitaxel (T)—the most common chemotherapy used to treat breast cancer— is . . . wait for it . . . derived from the Pacific yew tree. It took several years to isolate it in its pure form. It then took a considerable amount of time to study it, prove it worked, and make it into a drug that could be administered to a human. Let's put this into perspective. The first bark sample was collected by the USDA in 1962 as part of a specific push to develop medications from plants. Trials in humans started in 1984, and it was approved for breast cancer use in 1994. To date, it is the best-selling cancer drug ever manufactured, with annual peak sales in 2000 at $1.6 billion.

Words from Your Sisters:

You are not alone!

This was one of the hardest parts of the journey, the decision making part. You need to take a deep breath, get the information, and then make a decision talking with people you trust and love.

Survivor Sister

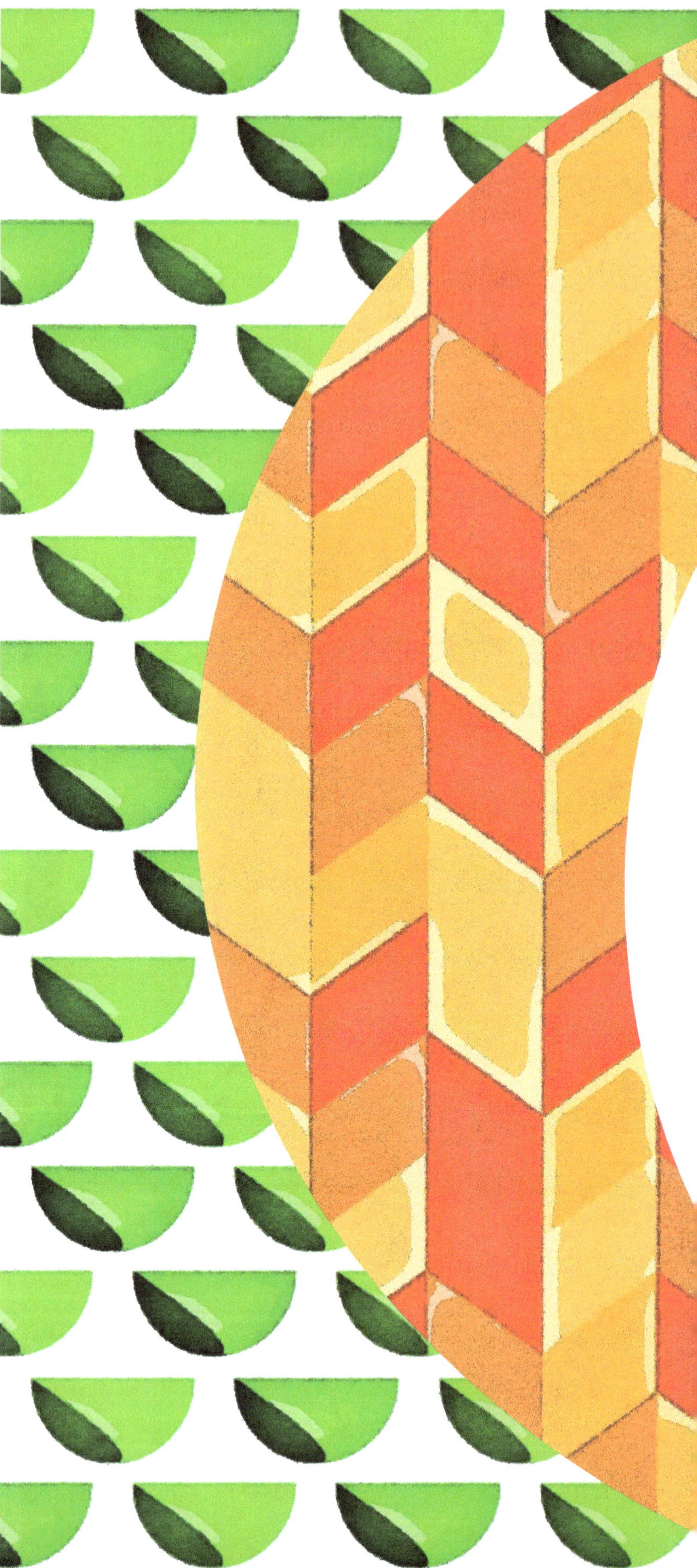

Genetics

Who Am I Really?

So you ended up with some not-so-desirable traits from Mom and Dad. (Yes, breast cancer genes can come from Dad too.) But did they unsuspectingly give you a higher risk of cancer? Maybe.

First, do you actually want to get genetic testing? Do you want to know? It's the Pandora's Box that you cannot close. And it's very personal. There used to be (and still are) a long list of criteria for getting tested. However, in 2019, the American Society of Breast Surgeons decided that all ladies with breast cancer should be given the option for testing. An important side note here is that not all insurance companies have jumped on this bandwagon yet. Genetics is a growing area of medicine, and increasingly, genetic testing is being recommended for people with cancer. Let's pro and con this one.

Pro: This is some powerful information that can help you make some serious decisions regarding your breast cancer care (think mastectomy vs. lumpectomy). Health insurance companies cannot discriminate against you because of your genetics; you can still get coverage (it's the law!). This information may just save your life! Suppose you are found to be at a higher risk of breast cancer, ovarian cancer, or colon cancer. If that's the case, it's time to take action! You just may live longer (think of interventions like screening colonoscopies and prophylactic surgeries). You can tell your family members, and you just may save their lives! A pathogenic genetic variant isn't just "bad news"; this is powerful news! People can start earlier and more intensive screening protocols. And while more frequent colonoscopies don't sound like fun, they could save a life! Or help someone you love find cancer earlier, at a lower stage, which could mean skipping therapies like chemo.

Con: You can't put the cat back in the bag; now you know! Also, unlike the nondiscrimination laws regarding health insurance, life insurance companies and disability insurance companies can't look the other way on this one. Yes, they can legally discriminate against you! But (sorry sister . . . newsflash) a cancer diagnosis has already changed your life insurance options. Another thing to consider is how your family members will react. You may totally freak out your family members who don't want the stress of knowing that they may be at increased risk (especially if they have young children, this can be scary stuff).

Genetic testing is still pretty new stuff in the grand scheme of things. It's going to be changing, and rapidly, for quite a long time. A negative test doesn't mean that you don't have a variant or mutation (necessarily). It could just be that we don't yet know about the genetic variant that you and your family have.

Also, please remember that it's your body. A genetic mutation doesn't mean that you now have to do anything. It also doesn't mean that you *have* to do something now (meaning that you may want to wait until you are done having babies). But, we do have some useful information to help guide you. For example, you could be told that your survival is greater if you have your breasts and ovaries removed.

Also, skip back to page 50 for a refresher on some genetics information that you were introduced to earlier!

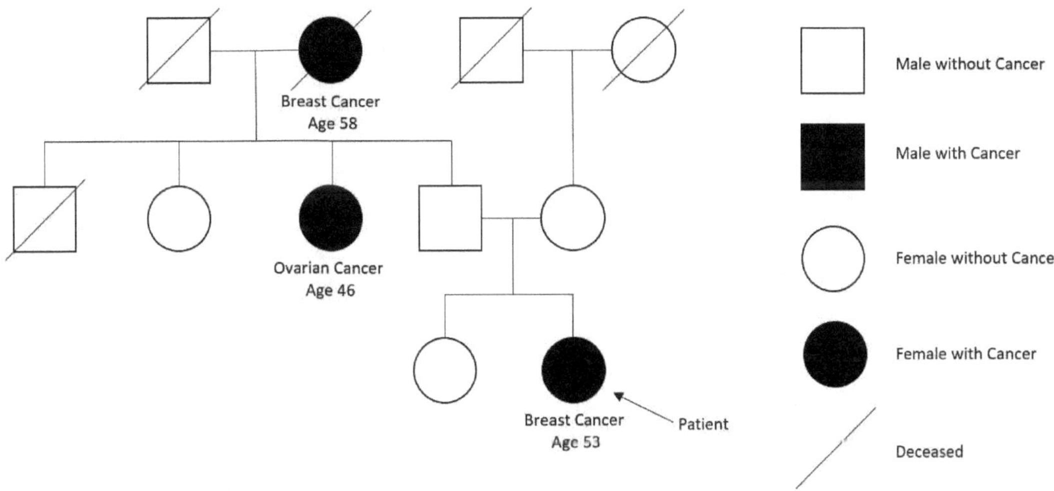

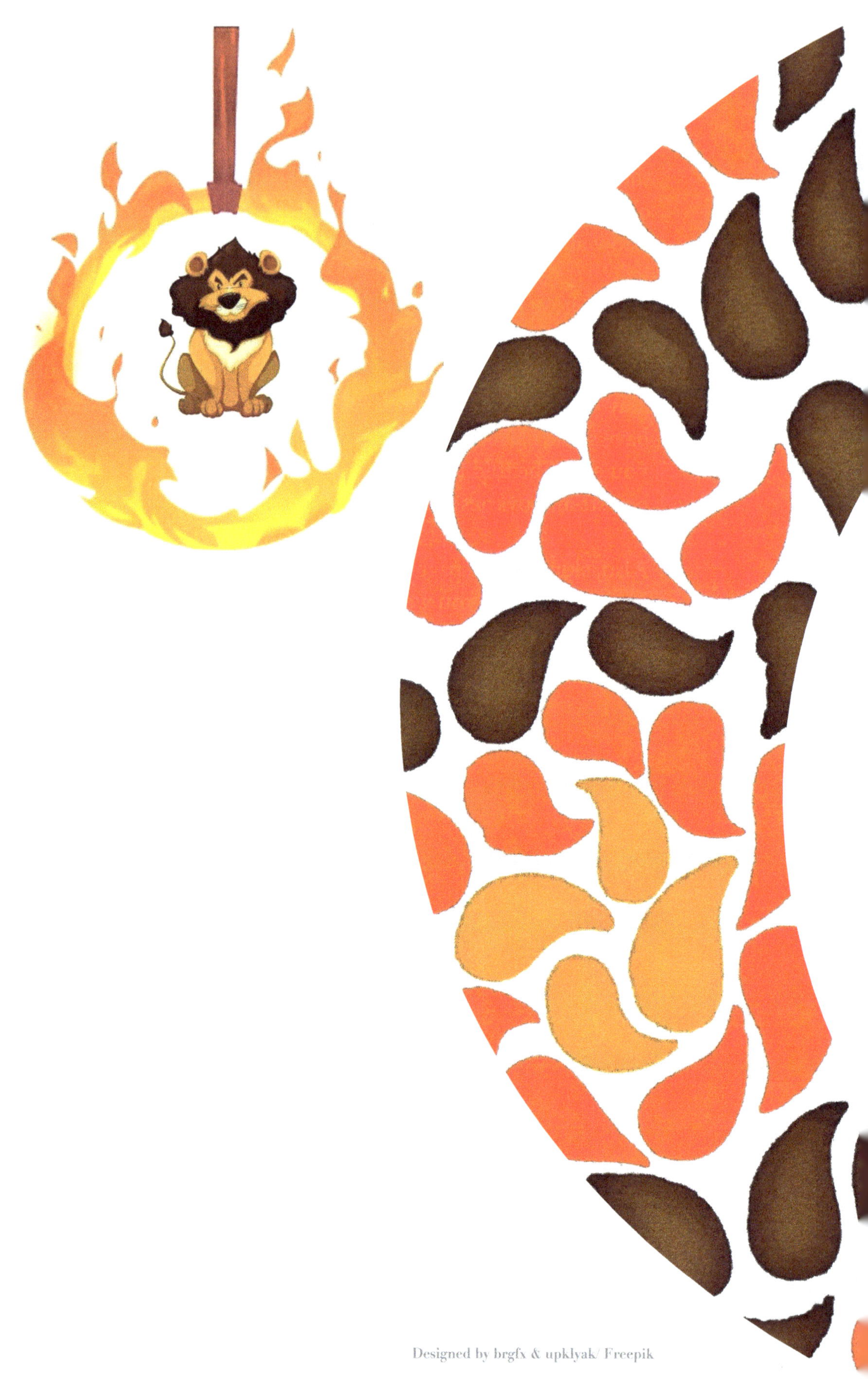

Survivorship

I Jumped Through Fire, Tamed Lions . . .

Finally, you are on the other side of all this. You've endured weeks, or months, or the better part of a year undergoing treatment. After the surgery, chemo, and radiation are finished you may be starting an anti-estrogen pill. Congrats, you made it! You may feel tired, accomplished, different, or relatively unchanged. We all experience life differently. So now what?

Well, if you have one or more breasts left at the end of this journey, you are going to need to continue yearly mammograms. And don't forget just how important these are. Set a reminder or get them in your birthday month each year. If you are high risk, you will also need to continue or discuss starting high-risk surveillance options (i.e., breast MRI). Of course, your brain just thought, "Am I high risk?" Not necessarily. Getting breast cancer doesn't automatically push you into the high-risk screening breast MRI category, so ask your doc if this is for you. (They will use an online calculator of sorts to help make that decision.) Crazy, right?

If you have *no* breasts or reconstructed breasts, you do not need annual screening imaging. Ta-da! See you later mammograms! But you should meet with your surgeon annually for a breast exam for at least five years. Some women with implants opt for breast MRI every two years (an FDA recommendation to monitor implant status). Sometimes pathogenic genetic variant carriers (especially BRCA1 or 2) go this route and get breast MRIs every two years because they are at an increased risk of new breast cancers even after bilateral mastectomies. And everyone should be on the lookout for new lumps, bumps, nipple changes, or skin rashes. When something new pops up, call sooner rather than later, girlfriend!

"What else can I do? Do I need to start drinking green juices?"

Oh boy! How do we start to navigate the "after" phase of this whole mess? More importantly, how do we prevent this from happening again? Well, assuming you have completed all your recommended therapy (yay for you!), there are some things you can do! You are entering what we call the "survivorship" phase. There is a 263 page published NCCN (National Comprehensive Cancer Network) "General Survivorship Principles" document for reference. But if that seems like a bit much for your weekend reading plans, this is where I tell you to basically do all things that you already know you should be doing.

1. Get your annual screening mammogram if you still have breasts (redundant, yes, but I would be remiss if I didn't repeat this one). Follow up with your doctors and a primary care physician and get any tests, lab work, and imaging that is recommended to you.

2. Ask for help if something doesn't seem right. You are never alone, sister. Shortness of breath? Fatigue? Memory problems? Lymphedema? Sexual dysfunction or vaginal dryness? Anxiety? Depression? Pain? Vaccine recommendations? Grab a microphone and ask someone in

your care team. Please don't be shy; we don't want you to suffer in silence. We want to help, and we can help.

3. Healthy lifestyle . . . this is the "easier said than done" section, but it is important. The leading cause of death in cancer survivors is heart disease. And some of these interventions have also been shown to decrease cancer recurrence.

- Obtain or maintain a healthy weight.

- Be physically active (a minimum of 150 minutes each week, if physically able).

- Fifty percent of your diet should be plant-based (fruits, vegetables, and healthy grains). Limit sugar, processed food, and red meat intake. Ask to see a nutritionist if you need guidance.

- Minimize alcohol (one drink per day or less) and quit smoking.

- Get enough sleep.

- Be safe in the sun (take cover and wear SPF; you don't want skin cancer too).

- Supplement use is not recommended unless you have a proven deficiency. Save your money for something fun.

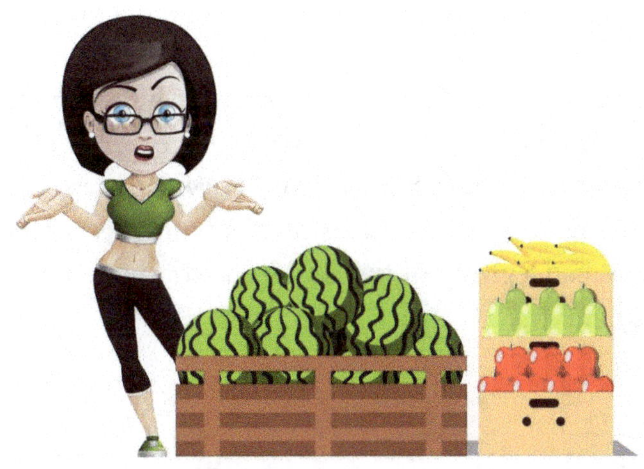

Surviving Breast Cancer

What To Do Next?

by DeBorrah Carter

I'm a survivor,
I'm not gon' give up
I'm not gon' stop,
I'm gon' work harder
I'm a survivor,
I'm gonna make it
I will survive,
keep on survivin'

~Destiny's Child, "Survivor" (2001)

Go on now, go, walk out the door
Just turn around now
'Cause you're not welcome anymore (DeBorrah adds "cancer you're not welcome anymore")
You think I'd crumble?
You think I'd lay down and die?
Oh no, not I, I will survive
Oh, as long as I know how to love, I know I'll stay alive . . .

Gloria Gaynor, "I Will Survive" (1978)

These two songs can be called "cancer mantras" for breast cancer survivors. Sure, they talk about love lost, and we certainly have no love lost for breast cancer. Yet the power of "I Will Survive" or "Survivor" resounds through the refrains. (I sang the Destiny's Child version at a women's conference six weeks after treatment and had a group of five hundred women standing on their feet, singing along with me.)

"Thank you, God, I survived breast cancer! Now what's next?"

You've come through diagnosis. You made it through treatment, whether it's surgery, chemotherapy, radiation, a combination of all, or maybe just one or two. But you made it through. Now what do you do? I'm a survivor and peer/patient breast cancer navigator. I know what I needed, so I'm sharing some of that knowledge with you.

Have a Survivorship Plan.

A survivorship plan is actually a folder in which you will have listed everything someone who cares for you will have access to (HIPPA approved). Keep it easily accessible so your "support team" can actually be your support team.

> In your survivorship plan will be the name(s) of all of your doctors, including your primary care physician, who is part of your "follow-up" team, as well as a nutritionist.
>
> List the medications you will be taking, including supplements (if allowed).
>
> Appointment dates and times, so your HIPPA approved caregiver can take you should you become unable drive yourself. If possible, always have someone with you during your visits. Note: Keep every appointment with your physicians. Some oncologists will follow you for five years. Some will follow you even longer. Try to find an oncologist who will be with you for a very long time and who listens to you.
>
> Log in all of your physician comments. Doing so will assist you and your caregiver as well as other doctors to know each step of your journey and allows them to better provide your aftercare needs.
>
> Your support team includes caregivers, trusted friends, other survivors, and a positive support group (if you have a group that you attend).

Each person on your team should be a positive individual. If there is someone who is toxic, negative, or always saying they are worried, then do not include them in your team, even if that person is a family member or close friend.

What your food preferences are. This is important because some of us have allergies or may not be able to tolerate certain foods because of medications. Some aftercare medications may give you hot flashes, so jot down what foods make you feel better.

A section for what makes you feel good (physically, mentally, and emotionally) and what makes you feel not so good. (This is not a replacement for your journal; however, your physicians need to know this information to help with any necessary adjustments, including medications and foods or activities.)

Love Yourself.

What do you mean, love myself? I mean just that. You are a "new you." Take care of yourself first, and don't try to do what everyone else feels you should. Relax, Rest, Release! You don't need to run a marathon during your first year of recovery. If you'd like to do a 5K walk, do it, but you don't have to. You don't need to become Martha Stewart. Enjoy meals that someone else prepares, or if you'd like to try some new recipe, do it, but not for fifty people. Do it just for yourself. Mind how you feel, not anyone else. Have someone give you a massage or just bask in the sunlight. Take a walk in the park. If you live in an area where you can see the stars, look out at night and be grateful for the beauty of the sky.

Keep a Greatfulness Journal.

Journals are wonderful in expressing yourself. Every day, find something to be grateful for. Every day, find one positive thing in spite of all the mess. Be grateful that even though you don't feel like getting out of bed, you have a bed. Even if you hate running to the restroom, you have a restroom. Find one thing every day.

Give Yourself a Makeover.

Are you out of your mind? A makeover? What? Yes, a makeover. You can do it! Personal story. My daughter lives 2300 miles away from me. She's a hairstylist. She flew to California and made me three beautiful wigs that could only fit my head. I had a "grocery store wig" for everyday activities. I had a "sassy wig" for those days I wanted to be sassy and stylish. Then she made me a "glamour wig" for those days I wanted to be sexy. Many hospitals can recommend wig specialists, if you so choose. I love hats, being originally from the East Coast. When I wasn't feeling a wig, I wore the most amazing hats—not just caps but real hats, even a leather cowgirl hat, along with some leather pants. I also love headwraps. I purchase the most beautiful (and still inexpensive) wraps, and they are very chic. YouTube has great videos for those who have never wrapped before.

Care for your skin! Speak with a certified cancer dermatologist or aesthetician about skin care.

Wear lipstick or lip gloss, even during a pandemic when no one can see your lips. You will feel better.

Lost your eyelashes? Okay. Just use a little eyeliner. For eyebrows, there are so many new products to make wonderful eyebrows and not come out looking like Joan Crawford! Need help? Ask someone you trust on your support team.

Get new lingerie! What? I had a mastectomy! I had a lumpectomy! What new lingerie? Are you crazy? I'm not feeling that one! Let me tell you, whether you have a prosthesis (or not) or breasts of different sizes, brand new lingerie will do wonders. Once again, many hospitals will be able to recommend you to a bra specialist or bra retailers who specialize in breast cancer. Get pretty stuff; it's out there. Get that trusted support friend to go with you or wade through online catalogs with you. If you have a cancer support group, make it a party. We are celebrating having another day of life! Another day . . . that is to be celebrated. I won't share my age here, but trust me, as a twenty-year survivor, I'm no spring chicken. But I love pretty bras and panties, even though no one but myself sees them. Can I get an amen, sister?

Acknowledge Your Fear.

We are all afraid that first year, or the next three years, and finally wondering if we will get to the magical number of five-year survivorship. Acknowledge it. It's okay to cry and share it with that trusted "support" person or write it in your journal or share it through CaringBridge, which is an online support group who may not know you personally but will give you a safe haven to share your feelings.

Surround Yourself with Loving People and Pray Together.

Live life! Find the most fun people you can and laugh, a lot. I have a friend that will call me up and say "Girl, let me tell you." She's a gossip, but I love her funny gossip stories. Not bad stuff, just funny stuff that she sees and calls to tell me. I'm a spiritual person, but not everyone is. I know and acknowledge Who brought me through this. I celebrated twenty years as a breast cancer survivor in February 2021. With all that I've written in this article, I could not have done it without God. I know that. For you, find that peace that surpasses all understanding and trust me. You will sing as I did "I'm a survivor. I'm gonna make it!"

Written by DeBorrah Carter, Sassy Survivor©, 20 years survivor. Used by permission, March 2021

Thoughts

Words from Your Sisters:

You are not alone!

I focused on research, well into the night sometimes. I found very little about the chemo hair loss experience. There is a lot written about the psychological effect, but the cold hard facts about what color does hair grow back, does taking an estrogen blocker effect the hair thickness when it regrows, what about coloring your hair. Nothing. So I went on a mission to get a research project going. It took several years of trials to find the right team. I have a great team now!

Survivor Sister

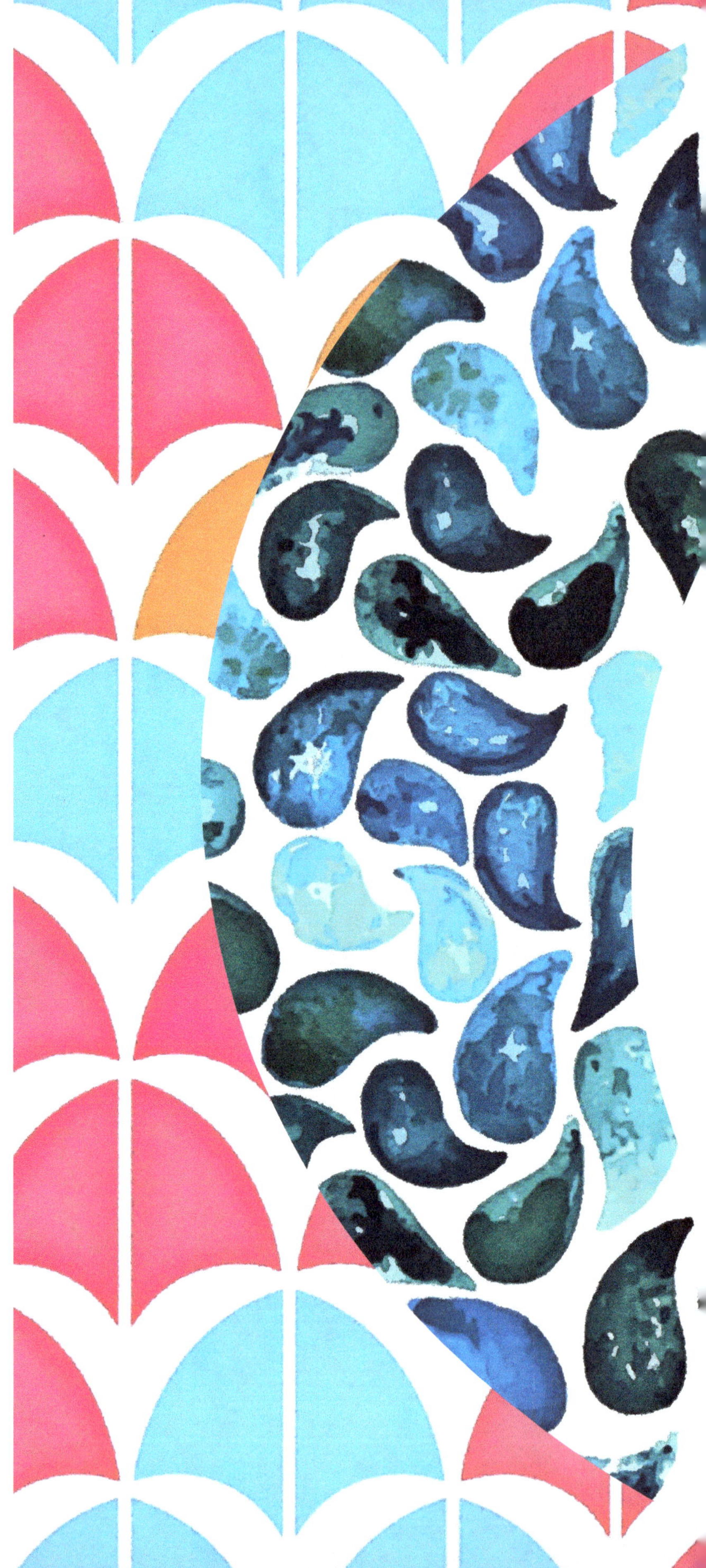

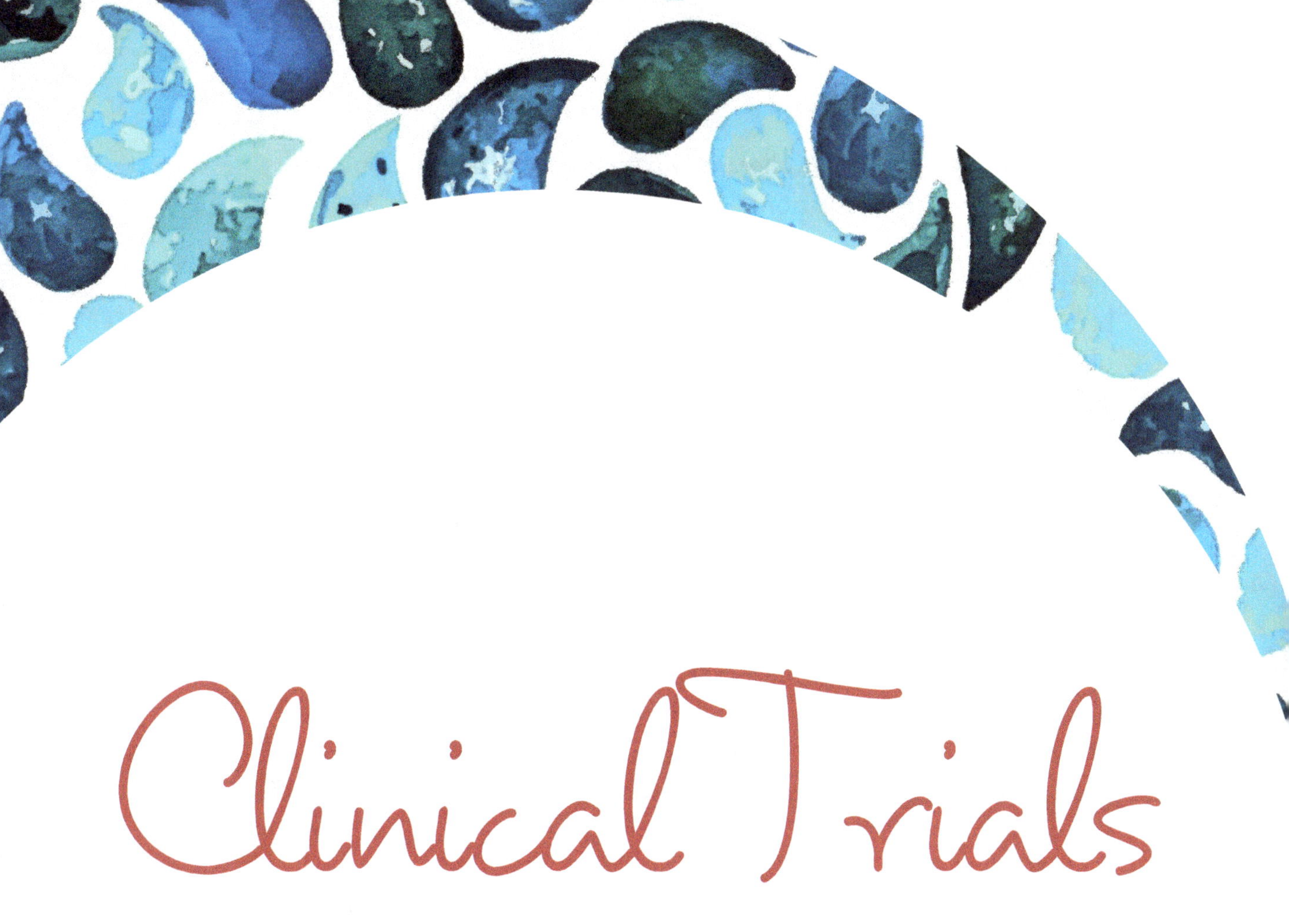

Clinical Trials

Do I Need One?

You may be offered participation in a clinical trial, or you may be counseled to seek out a clinical trial depending on a whole host of factors! You are probably not thinking, Wow, this is just too easy! I need something more complex to ponder. But, hold on a sec! Clinical trials are fantastic!

Clinical trials will usually put you at the cutting-edge of new science (think medications that you would not otherwise have access to), they can have their perks (think free imaging), and they can sometimes change your surgery plan (like less surgery in those armpits, which translates to less risk of lymphedema). That's right! There are clinical trials ongoing to change how we do surgery, change how we give chemotherapy, investigate new medications, and change how we give radiation.

There is always room for improvement, right? Remember, we got "here" because of the thousands of women that went before you and took that leap of faith and some extra time and testing to gift you your current options. Take a moment of thanks for these trailblazing women and their dedicated doctors and scientists. It is only because of clinical trials that sentinel lymph nodes and breast conservation are an option! Without change and advancement, we would still be performing radical mastectomies on everyone.

I know some of you are thinking, I am no lab rat! Give me the "tried and true," doc! But, by design, clinical trials have a ton of safety checks to minimize potential risks to you. Clinical trials are rolled out in a few phases, and each phase has a specific goal. Remember, new medications have gone through a rigorous preclinical evaluation before they are offered to a person.

Here's a quick rundown of the phases a new medication must go through before it becomes our new "tried and true" for the next generation.

> Phase 0: How does this new drug work in the human body? A small amount of the drug is given to ten to fifteen people.
>
> Phase 1: What's a good dose with low side effects? Fifteen to thirty people are enrolled.
>
> Phase 2: Okay, so it seems safe, but is it really safe? This phase focuses on a specific type of cancer. It is given in combination with other proven drugs with the continued goal to monitor for safety (given to a larger group of people).
>
> Phase 3: Looks safe! Now let's see how it stacks up to the competition (the competition being the standard therapy at that time). More than one hundred people are enrolled, and this is when a process called

randomization is usually introduced. Meaning that if you agree to the trial, you are randomly assigned to a study group. There are usually two or more study groups. One group, the "control" group, gets the standard of care. (You aren't getting anything more or less than you would be getting outside of the trial.) This group will set the bar for the other group. In contrast, the other group or groups receives the standard of care with a new medication added. This will all depend on the study design, and research nurses will be there to explain it all!

Phase 4: This phase starts after the drug is FDA approved and is in use. It is the continuous monitoring of a drug once it becomes available to the broader public. Again, the aim is for safety. A drug may not show rare side effects during the first three phases. But, if 1 in 10,000 people experience a particular side effect, it will be picked up here.

Remember that if you decline study participation, there is no love lost between you and your care team. It is perfectly fine to do whatever is right for you. Also remember that you don't have to seek out a trial as part of your cancer care. Trials have stringent criteria for participation, and you may not fit those criteria.

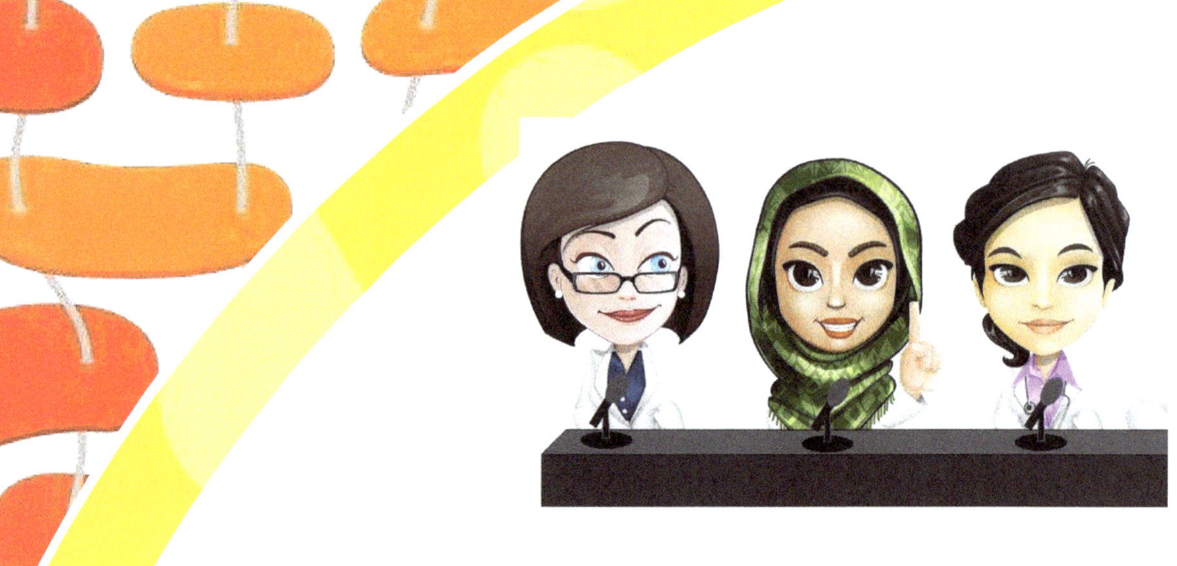

Do I Need a Second Opinion? Or a Third?

Sometimes finding the right doctor is more about a good match between two people (you and the doc) than simply seeking out the most convenient or most highly recommended specialist. You need to feel comfortable putting that person on your team and seeing them for many, many years. Also, you need to feel confident in the plan. If the

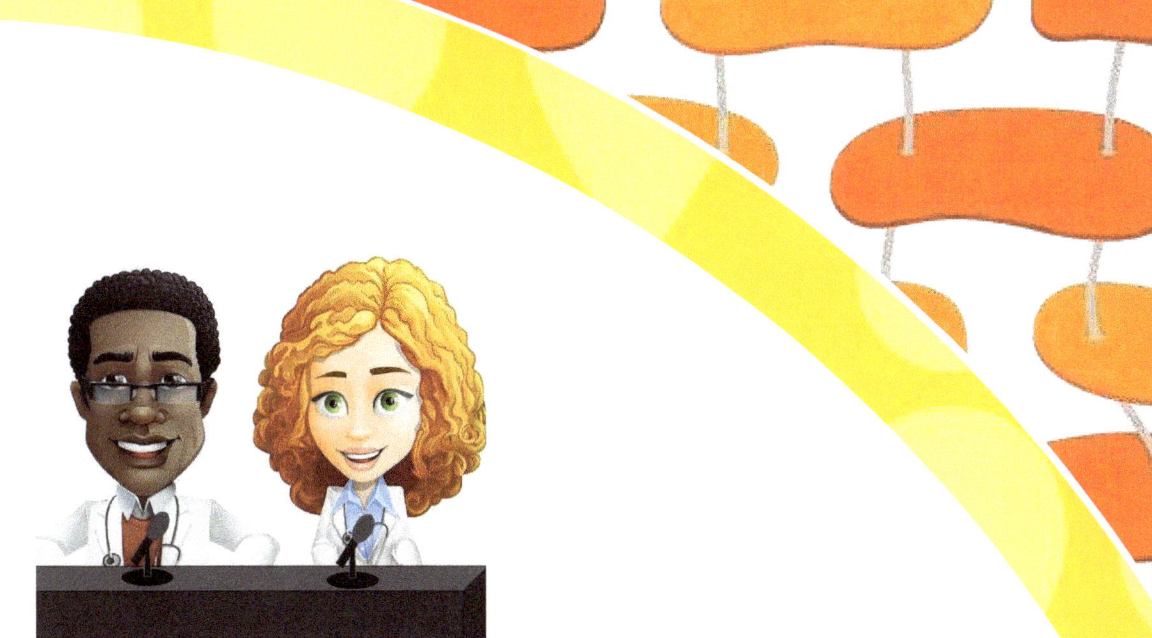

first doc you go to doesn't fit the bill, then find another doc! Confirm your treatment options.

It's your body and your life; be your own advocate and do what you need to do. Doctors are not offended by second opinions. That being said, if you find yourself "doctor shopping" for the doc that will tell you what you want to hear and do only what you want to do . . . knock it off! Here's an example to highlight this scenario: You want to keep your nipples, period! But you have been to two or three surgeons who say your cancer involves the nipple, and there is no safe way to save the nipple and perform a nipple-sparing mastectomy. If you are making an appointment to see yet another surgeon, take a moment to pause and consider the possibility that nipple-sparing mastectomy is not an option for you. You need to stop dragging your heels and delaying your cancer care. Things do not always go how we want them to go (huge understatement, I know). Take a deep breath. You can do this!

Resources

I Need More!

Nccn.org
NCCN Guidelines are the rule book for cancer. They are updated every few years, so they aren't ever "outdated," but sometimes real life outpaces the rule book. They have links for patients so that you don't end up staring at a page of acronyms feeling totally overwhelmed.

Komen.org
The Susan G. Komen site has resources and can connect you to other women, marathons (yes, you will run again, or maybe for the first time!), and much more.

Most of the major cancer centers (hospitals that only do cancer care), academic institutions (affiliated with a college), and the major hospital systems have a breast cancer resource page. The good and bad thing about cancer is that it happens to so many women that you will not be at a loss for information. The bad news is that there is *so* much information! My word of advice? Get off the computer. There is some scary stuff and there is some hopeful stuff, but it is damn hard to sort out what part of this whole mess applies to you. The spectrum of breast cancer runs from something analogous to run-of-the-mill skin cancer (not bad) to pancreatic cancer (very bad). It's an umbrella term that really doesn't do it justice when you are trying to sort through the Googled rubble. So stop. Ask some experts, get a second opinion if you need it in order to sleep at night. Then move along with making plans and living life.

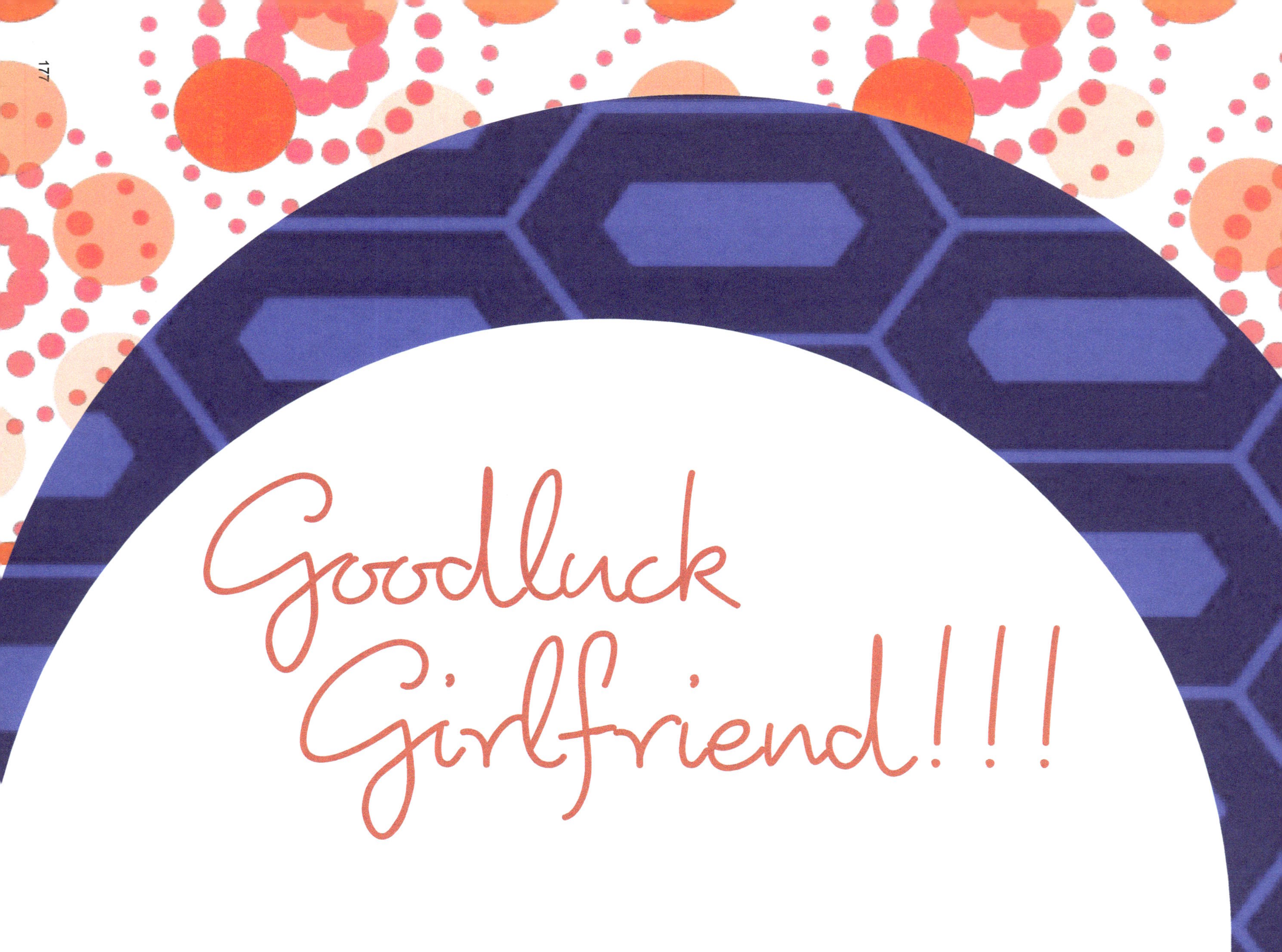
Goodluck
Girlfriend!!!

You Can Do This!

Show up for all those darn appointments. Don't forget to keep on living and enjoying life. If you are feeling overwhelmed, figure out what the next step is and focus on that —only that. Forget the rest. Baby steps, fierce lady. You can do this!

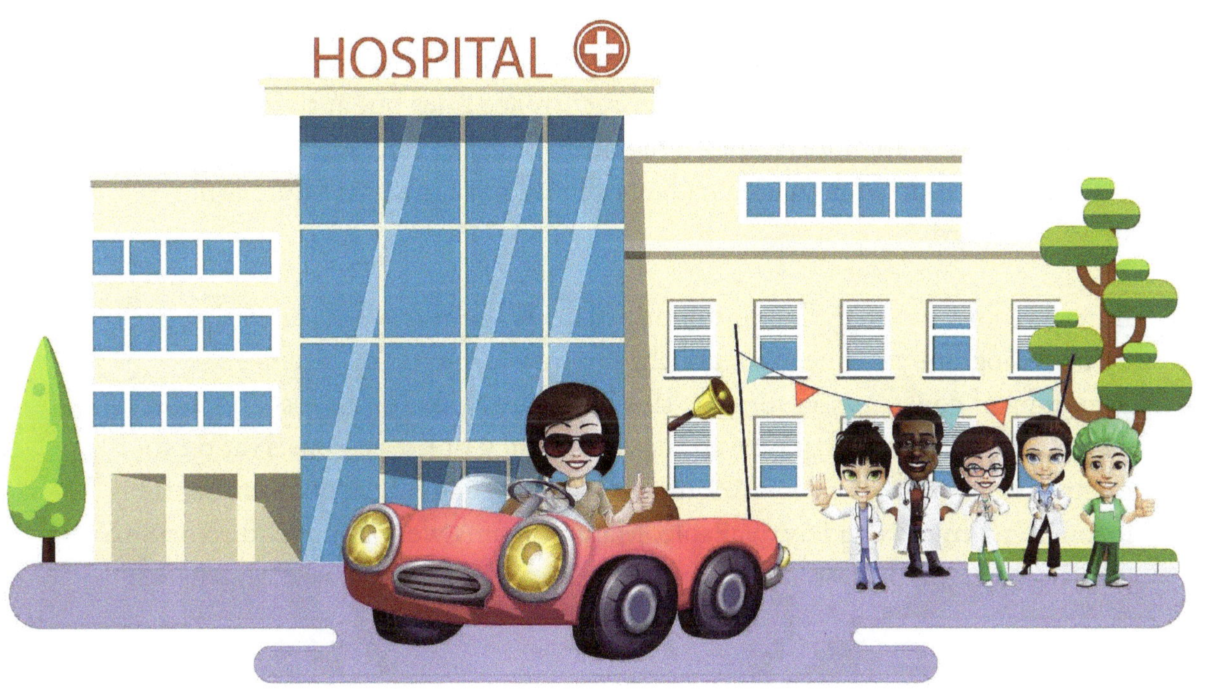

Expert Extras

In Case You Needed a Little More . . .

"A Detailed and Debated Debrief on MRI"

by Dr. Alan Hollingsworth

One of the most difficult challenges in successful breast cancer surgery is the avoidance of local recurrence. While the medical oncologists are monitoring the rest of the body, the breast surgeon and radiation oncologist oversee eradicating the tumor locally. That said, there is considerable controversy surrounding the best way to achieve low local recurrence rates.

Taking a larger amount of normal tissue around the tumor site as part of the lumpectomy specimen will offer lower recurrence rates but at the cost of a worse cosmetic outcome. Adding a radiation boost to the lumpectomy site works, too, but deciding which patients should have this extra dose is not straightforward.

Enter preoperative mapping of tumor extent. While it is often stated that pre-op mammography has been part of the "lumpectomy package" since the beginning of conservation surgery, this is not the case. The largest and most definitive clinical trial that proved the equivalency of breast conservation to mastectomy (the NSABP B-06, launched in 1976) actually took place before mammography was widely available. Mammograms were not a requirement to participate in the B-06 study, nor were outcomes evaluated based on whether mammography had been performed. The presence or absence of pre-op mammography was simply recorded in a large database. Given the B-06 design, one can argue that relatively good breast conservation surgery can be performed without any type of pre-op imaging. Yet, recurrence rates at the lumpectomy site were higher in the B-06 trial than what patients face today.

Nevertheless, as breast conservation became widely adopted, no one questioned the benefit of pre-op mammography as providing a road map for the surgeon in women who had not been diagnosed by screening mammography already—that is, "diagnostic mammography" for those women presenting with palpable tumors became the norm. Later, ultrasound was added in some cases to evaluate dense breast tissue and to determine if lymph nodes required needle biopsy before surgery.

When breast magnetic resonance imaging (MRI) was introduced to the clinic in the early 2000s, it was clear that mammography was missing additional sites of tumor. Three benefits of MRI were proposed: 1) improved accuracy of the lumpectomy technique used; 2) detection of cancers located in the same breast, but at a separate site, and 3) detection of cancers in the opposite breast. At the same time, critics asked whether finding these additional sites of cancer altered results above and beyond mammography alone.

The clinical impact of pre-op MRI is more likely to be found in #2 and #3 above. But instead of focusing on these separate (unknown) cancers that might be inadequately treated without MRI, the controversy focused almost entirely on the lumpectomy site. MRI was alleged by some to lower the positive margin rate and/or the local recurrence rate, while others saw no benefit. In the end, a large combined study indicated no measurable benefit as far as the lumpectomy site goes.

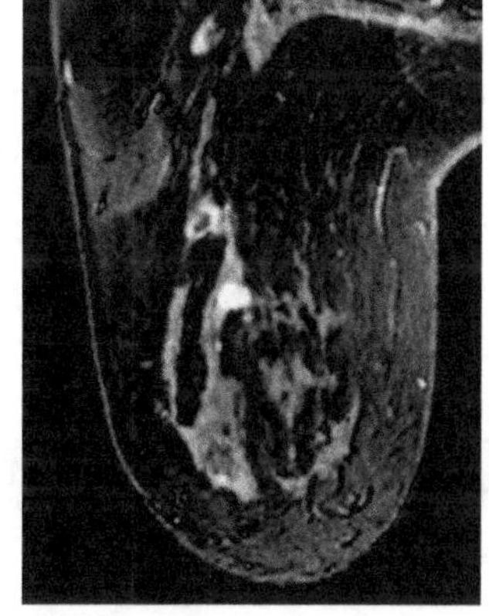

Breast MRI
Courtesy of
Dr. Alan Hollingsworth

The downside of MRI has always been the "false-positive" problem wherein completely benign entities might prompt the radiologist to perform extra biopsies. Since this problem was a "given," the benefit of MRI had to be clearly demonstrated. That said, centers of excellence focused heavily on minimizing the false-positive rate, prompting a large variation in published results, some institutions showing a benefit to pre-op MRI, others not.

The question at hand was not simply the miss-rate of mammography, a well-documented problem in those studies where breast MRI was used for asymptomatic screening of high-risk patients (with MRI doubling or tripling the rate of detected cancers). No, the challenge went deeper than that. The critics of MRI wanted to know how long-term outcomes were altered by discovering these extra cancers being missed on mammography. That's a more difficult question to answer than simply counting cancers found on MRI.

Granted, the secondary cancers on the same side as the known cancer were usually small when discovered on MRI, likely handled by the combination of systemic therapies plus whole breast radiation. But then, a new approach to radiation emerged, where only the lumpectomy site was irradiated. This opened the controversy of additional sites of cancer once again when realizing that these second (or even third) tumors were not going to be incidentally irradiated as one sees when the entire breast is irradiated. Instead, with the radiation target being the lumpectomy site alone, these additional tumors would be essentially untreated (though there is some local benefit with chemo and/or endocrine agents).

So, how often are these second (or third) sites of cancer present in the same breast, invisible on mammography? The probabilities are relatively small, keeping the fires of controversy well lit. For instance, in our experience of 2,000 consecutive pre-op breast MRIs, 3 percent of women had distinct secondary tumors at a site distant to the known primary on the same side. This small group of patients can easily have "clear margins" around the primary tumor because the unknown cancer is so far away, thus giving a false sense of security.

Another 4 percent had extensive disease seen on MRI involving multiple quadrants of the breast, prompting mastectomy in all such cases. Here, without

MRI, the patients will eventually get the correct treatment, but only after multiple trips to the operating room trying to get clear margins for a cancer growth pattern where the MRI could have told the surgeon upfront: "Don't even try for clear margins. It will not be possible."

And what about the other breast? Nearly everyone has agreed that cancer will be discovered in the opposite breast in 3 to 4 percent of newly diagnosed patients (similar to the cancer yield in high-risk screening patients). However, the significance of this relatively small number is hotly debated. Critics of pre-op breast MRI point out that these missed cancers on the opposite side are usually early stage and low grade, unlikely to increase breast cancer mortality if simply left alone and discovered later through mammography or by palpation.

Yet, we argued from our series that one-half of the discoveries on the opposite side were the same stage or worse stage than the known primary. This was demonstrated most dramatically when the known primary was non-life-threatening DCIS, while the MRI-discovered cancer on the opposite side was invasive breast cancer. While this occurred in only 2 percent of DCIS patients, the implication is powerful—in essence, without MRI, if the patient opts for lumpectomy for her known DCIS, the life-threatening cancer remains in the patient on the opposite side, untreated (tamoxifen or other endocrine agents might help, but are not curative alone). The tough question is this: Do you perform pre-op MRI in 100 patients to find the two who benefit, while at the same time, twenty-five will be called back for extra study, and ten will have a benign biopsy as a result of pre-op MRI? It's easy to see why pre-op MRI is controversial.

A major contribution to this controversy is the fact that different institutions publish widely different experience. As a result, the American Society of Breast Surgeons most recently stated that pre-op MRI should not be considered as a routine part of the pre-operative work-up. That does not mean a moratorium on pre-op MRI, but implies the need to use the tool selectively, primarily in women with dense breasts and/or lobular histology where growth patterns and separate tumor sites can be difficult to see on mammography.

Preoperative MRI can have an entirely different use in more advanced stages of breast cancer wherein the order of events is reversed, and chemotherapy is delivered up front (neoadjuvant) rather than following surgery. The question in all patients undergoing pre-op neoadjuvant therapy is whether the chosen chemotherapy regimen is working. Physical exam alone over the course of several months of pre-op chemotherapy can be misleading as tumors can remain palpable even when there are no living cells within. Thus, there has been extensive research on breast imaging methods to determine a better way of evaluating the efficacy of the chemotherapy regimen being utilized.

Of the various imaging methods available, it appears that breast MRI is the most accurate way to assess whether chemotherapy is working. If it is not working, the regimen can be changed. On the other hand, when the chemo is successfully doing its job, a shrinking tumor on a follow-up MRI brings up two possibilities: 1) any tumor cells that escaped the breast before diagnosis are likely being destroyed as well, and thus a better prognosis overall for the patient, and 2) some women who are not lumpectomy candidates due to large tumor size can be "converted" to lumpectomy candidacy after successful pre-operative (adjuvant) chemotherapy. Breast MRI performed both before and after chemo—rather than relying on palpation, mammography or ultrasound—is the best method to follow progress. However, it remains true that the only definitive way to measure the full impact of chemotherapy is when the pathologist is looking at the treated tissue under the microscope.

"Lymphedema"

by Dr. Lisa Spiguel

Say yes to quality of life! Through the years, there has been a shift toward focusing on the quality of life. This is because patients survive breast cancer. Yes, in the US, it is estimated that 3.4 million women live with a personal history of breast cancer. Even though breast cancer incidence remains stable, mortality continues to decline due to early detection, advances in systemic therapy, as well as breast cancer outreach and education. Statistics demonstrate that, of women diagnosed in 2020, 90 percent of them will be alive in five years. This is awesome! We need to focus not only on advancing our understanding of breast cancer treatment but also on understanding what we can do to improve the overall quality of life of our breast cancer survivors.

This brings to light lymphedema, which continues to remain one of the side effects related to breast cancer treatment. Lymphedema is most affected by the extent of surgery on the breast and lymph nodes, the need for radiation to the breast, chest, and lymph nodes, the need for certain chemotherapy agents, as well as body composition, with women with higher body weight at higher risk for lymphedema. The reason arm lymphedema occurs is because the lymph nodes under the arm, or what we call the axillary lymph nodes, are important lymph nodes for both the breast and the arm. Therefore, when we, as clinicians, remove them or treat them with radiation therapy or prescribe certain chemotherapy agents, we can affect the function of the lymph nodes and lymphatic channels, which ultimately leads to the back up of fluid in the arm—or lymphedema. The lymphatic system is a complex network of channels in the body that is responsible for bringing fluid back to the circulation when an injury occurs or when a person has an infection. The lymph nodes are little round or oval structures that redirect the fluid from the lymph channels of the body into the circulatory system and are also important in presenting infections as well as tumor cells to the body so that the body's immune system can fight infection or help defeat cancer.

As stated previously, the biggest risks of lymphedema are surgery, radiation, chemotherapy, and body habitus. Let's start with surgery. The bigger the operation on the breast and lymph nodes, the bigger the risk. Although data shows that mastectomy has a higher risk of arm lymphedema than breast-saving surgery, the bigger the surgery on the lymph nodes is the greatest risk. Over the years, we, as clinicians, have found ways to sample the lymph nodes rather than just removing all of the lymph nodes under the arm. The sampling procedure is known as "sentinel lymph node biopsy." This procedure is used for women whose lymph nodes do not appear to be involved with cancer both on examination as well as on imaging. The procedure allows us to find the first draining lymph nodes of the breast. On average, there are between one to five lymph nodes, and these lymph nodes act as the gatekeeps of the other axillary lymph nodes. If they are negative for cancer spread, then the risk of additional axillary lymph nodes being involved with cancer is exceedingly low. This technique became the standard of care for women with clinically normal lymph nodes in the late 1990s and early 2000s.

Why it is important to focus on sentinel lymph node biopsy is that sentinel lymph node biopsy has a much lower risk of lymphedema than the routine removal of all axillary lymph nodes. Numerous studies demonstrate the risk of lymphedema with sentinel lymph node biopsy to be under 8 percent, as compared to doing more comprehensive surgery on the lymph nodes called axillary lymph node dissection. Lymphedema rates with axillary lymph node dissection have been shown to be as high as 40 percent in some studies. Therefore, over the years, we have challenged the use of sentinel lymph node biopsy alone in patients who are clinically node-negative as well as patients who undergo breast-saving surgery and have a very small amount of lymph node metastasis on pathology evaluation. Strong data supports the use of sentinel lymph node biopsy alone in these groups of patients, demonstrating no difference in survival from breast cancer as well as no difference in recurrence, which is the risk that cancer can come back. We have even used this procedure alone in patients who have lymph nodes involved at the time of diagnosis, who undergo chemotherapy prior to surgery, and their lymph nodes become negative following chemotherapy treatment, but prior to their operation. So, it is important to discuss these options with your treating surgeon to see if you are a candidate for sentinel lymph node biopsy alone or maybe a candidate to avoid lymph node surgery all together.

However, some patients need to have all of their axillary lymph nodes removed or an axillary lymph node dissection. The number of lymph nodes removed is really individual to each patient and is also affected by whether a patient has undergone chemotherapy prior to surgery. However, an axillary lymph node dissection is needed in some patients. There are options though. When axillary lymph node dissection is needed, there are specialized techniques available at some institutions to reduce the risk of lymphedema, such as lymph venous bypass. This technique uses a similar concept of sentinel lymph node biopsy, however, it places the dye in the arm rather than the breast to find the lymphatic channels that are important for the arm. Following removal of the axillary lymph nodes, the surgeon, typically a microsurgeon, finds the lymphatic channels of the arm and re-routes them into an available vein so that those lymphatic channels do not scar off and can remain open and draining into the circulation, even after removal of the lymph nodes. Studies have demonstrated that with this procedure, the lymphedema rate can be as low as 5 percent. There are also clinical trials available at institutions throughout the country to determine whether we can safely save the lymph nodes of the arm if they aren't found to be important to the breast. This is the Alliance 221702 Trial, Axillary Reverse Mapping. This trial hopes to change the way we surgeons perform axillary node dissection so that we can do so in a way to minimize lymphedema risk while maintaining cancer treatment.

Radiation therapy is also one of the leading risk factors to developing lymphedema, and studies support the combination of removing all axillary lymph nodes plus the addition of radiation therapy to be the biggest risk. There has been active attention in this arena so that we as clinicians do our best to minimize a double insult to the arm lymphatics. We as clinicians understand this risk and try to minimize the need for both axillary node dissection and radiation therapy. Clinical trials have demonstrated the safety in omitting axillary node dissection in certain women with minimal nodal disease, such as demonstrated in the US Trial ACOSOG Z0011, as well as additional international trials AATRM, IBCSG, AMAROS, and OTOASAR trials. We also have ongoing US clinical trials demonstrating the use of sentinel lymph node biopsy alone in women who undergo neoadjuvant chemotherapy for nodal disease and are found to have no residual disease following chemotherapy. As well as active US trial, Alliance 011202 Trial, evaluating who undergo sentinel lymph node biopsy following chemotherapy and are found to have small residual nodal disease on pathology. These trials are crucial in determining if sentinel lymph node biopsy is safe and whether radiation alone rather than in combination with surgery is successful.

I will touch lightly on chemotherapy risk, as this has been shown to be only a subset of chemotherapeutic agents and is thought to be mostly a transient risk, which means that it typically resolves after chemotherapy is ended. The agents notorious for leading to a temporary arm swelling are taxane agents, such as docetaxel and paclitaxel. The agents have demonstrated a potential effect on the ability of the lymph channels to contract or push fluid towards the lymph nodes. Although the studies demonstrated that swelling that may develop typically resolves following treatment. So, if you notice that your arm appears heavier or swollen during chemotherapy, there is a chance that it can resolve following treatment.

Lastly, I will discuss the importance of a lymphedema surveillance team. If possible, it is very important to undergo evaluation by certified lymphedema specialists both prior to any treatment as well as following treatment. Measuring symptoms, arms circumference/volume measurements, lymph flow, as well as body composition are all important. Diagnosing lymphedema is a compilation of measurements, and many times, we as clinicians can find early signs of lymphedema prior to the patient noticing any change in their arm. This is important because finding signs of lymphedema prior to a patient noticing any change helps reduce the severity of lymphedema. An important part of the evaluation is also understanding your body composition, most importantly your body mass index or BMI. Many studies demonstrate elevated risks of lymphedema in women with higher body weights, with a three times higher risk of lymphedema in women with a BMI greater than thirty. Studies also demonstrate a decrease in lymphedema risk with decreasing your body weight. What is important exercise and diet for your heart health is the same as for your breast and lymphatic health. So be proactive and discuss with your treating team evaluation by physical therapy. Many institutions also have nutritionists available to counsel patients on developing a better diet.

Overall, we need to focus on the overall wellbeing of our breast cancer patients, and by understanding personal lymphedema risk and ways to minimize the risk is crucial!

"Bras and Prosthetics and Posture, Oh My!"

by Victoria Hand

As a Certified Mastectomy Fitter (CFM) with fifteen years of experience in the prosthetic industry, I hope to offer some helpful information on different options for breast prosthesis following a mastectomy or lumpectomy for breast cancer. A breast form helps to restore balance to your skeletal and muscular physiology. When natural weight is removed from your body, the body shifts to accommodate this lesser weight. In the case of a mastectomy, this shift can lead to rounded shoulders, poor posture, and neck pain. Of course, a prosthesis is not just physically important, it can also be helpful for emotional reasons. A breast prosthesis can help the patient to feel more like themselves and improve self-esteem.

Prostheses, also called breast forms, come in many sizes and shapes and are made from many different materials. The type of prosthesis needed following a mastectomy would be based on the surgical pattern. Some questions considered when choosing a prosthesis are, "Did the patient have a simple mastectomy? Were lymph nodes removed? Is the pectoralis major muscle intact?" Based on the answers to those questions, a 100 percent medical-grade silicone prosthesis would be selected. Traditional silicone forms come in full weight or lightweight medical grade silicone.

If the patient has had a unilateral mastectomy, measurements are taken to help determine which size and shape prosthesis is necessary to create symmetry. Prostheses are available in sizes 00–18. However, the numeric size will not be the only thing to consider. The remaining breast will also be measured to determine if a shallow, average, or full prosthetic is needed. The shape will be determined as well as color. The options for a prefabricated prosthesis are extensive, with over thirty different shapes available.

Shapers, also known as balancers or partials, are breast prostheses that are useful when the patient has had a lumpectomy and only needs a little bit of fullness to create symmetry.

A custom breast prosthesis is a great alternative for ladies who are undetermined about reconstructive surgery or have had a difficult time finding the right prefabricated prosthesis. A custom breast prosthesis is unique to a patient's size, shape, and surgical pattern and gives a more intimate and personalized fit to the chest wall. The custom prosthesis is fabricated following a 3D digital scan of the patient's remaining breast/surgical pattern. The state-of-the-art 3D scan has superior accuracy to guarantee a well-fitting prosthesis and is completely safe used by a multitude of prosthetic medical professionals. Following the scan, the prosthesis is then carefully designed, creating a personalized shape, natural appearance, and able to fit within any bra, not just mastectomy bras.

Also available following a mastectomy are lighter-weight prostheses that are great for swimming and exercising. The lightweight forms come in different materials, memory foam, fiberfill, and microbeads. These forms are great for offering the symmetric shape yet remaining cooler and drying faster (if used for swimming).

Frankly, the options are unlimited for patients that must undergo the scary diagnosis of breast cancer. It is so important to broaden awareness about options for breast prostheses. Finding a certified fitter will help provide the patient with the correct style of prosthesis to match her lifestyle, and for the prosthetist, there is nothing more rewarding than seeing a patient regain her confidence.

"Proton Therapy"
by Dr. David Schomas

"I want the best!"

Just as the technology we use day-to-day has changed dramatically, so, too, has the technology we use to treat breast cancer. Remember when phones were just for calling someone? Now there is a good chance you are using your phone to read this book!

Technological developments have clearly advanced care for patients with breast cancer, but at the same time, they have also created anxiety by creating options.

Numerous, well-done clinical trials have tested and evaluated radiation techniques, and advancement will continue. These studies are the results of motivated and dedicated patients partnering with institutions devoted to advancing breast cancer care. Just page through this book, or do a brief internet search, and it can quickly become overwhelming. It's daunting for patients to see so many different techniques, options, schedules, side effects, and outcomes. Options. Gone are the days of "Hello, my name is Dr. so-and-so, and this is what we are going to do." Today, the discussions around these options are lengthy, nuanced, and complicated.

Possibly the most obvious example of this progressing change is proton therapy . . . only one letter changes between photon and proton, but needless to say, it ain't that simple. Let's break it down so we all have an understanding of what proton therapy for breast cancer is and what it is not.

As we pointed out previously, radiation is either delivered externally (external beam radiation) or internally (brachytherapy). Let's focus again on the external beam technique.

There are three ways to deliver external beam radiation therapy.

Photons: Photons are considered the "traditional radiation treatment," and the vast majority of patients who receive, and who have received, external treatment receive photons. A photon is an "X-ray," which is part of the energy spectrum akin to light or radio waves. They do not have mass. (You will have to promise not to tell Albert Einstein or any other theoretical physicists that I told you photons don't have mass.) The photon energy can be adjusted in order to deposit dose at different depths in tissue. These invisible "energy packets" can be customized to meet a patient's very specific anatomy.

Electrons: Electrons are most often used in conjunction with photons to treat breast cancer. Unlike photons, electrons are actual particles, albeit very small particles, that do have mass. They "live" in the outside "cloud" region of an atom. Due in part to their small size, they do not penetrate tissue as deeply as photons. Depending on the patient and the treatment design needs, this can be advantageous.

Protons: Unlike photons, protons are actual particles that have mass and "live" inside the nucleus of an atom. Compared to electrons, they are huge! In fact, a proton is about 2,000 times heavier than an electron. Due to this larger weight, protons can be used to deposit dose "deeper" into tissue. Imagine a tennis ball being hit at nearly the speed of light at a target on the wall. Now imagine a 125-pound medicine ball at the gym being thrown at almost the same speed at the target. Actually, never mind; don't imagine that because I think it might create a black hole and end of all life on earth. But you get the idea. Protons are way bigger than electrons, and both are moving really, really fast.

So now that we have defined these three ways to deliver external beam radiation treatment, let us discuss a bit more about protons and photons.

For many decades, photon therapy has been utilized in cancer treatments. The photon has not changed. However, the technique and design, and the ability to shape, carve, customize and modulate photons has changed dramatically, allowing physicians to modify treatment planning. This has absolutely allowed for increased effectiveness of treatments with decreased toxicity. A phone call is still a phone call, but a modern smart phone is way different than a rotary wall phone, right?

In that context, enter the proton! Ta-da! Proton treatment! Proton therapy is new, right? Well, sorta. Back in the 1950s, it had a very niche role in treating certain cancers, available only at a few major cancer centers performing research. Over the decades, however, it has become more widely available throughout the country. The original promise of proton therapy for breast cancer was the potential to improve outcomes while decreasing toxicity. However, to date, despite intense and numerous efforts, no studies have shown this promise to be realized. All available information points to the equivalence of protons and photons in terms of both outcomes and side effects. So proton treatment is simply another way of delivering external beam therapy; it's another way to do the same thing.

As a radiation oncologist, I hear all the time, "I want the best. What is the best treatment?" It certainly can be confusing and overwhelming when patients hear that one therapy is better than another. There is an abundance of unfiltered information available on the internet and shared between friends and neighbors! It is very important to know there is no evidence that proton treatment is better than photon treatment. For this reason, the significant additional cost of proton therapy has made the delivery of proton treatment controversial. Because of this, many insurance companies will not cover the cost.

Proton or photon, radiation therapy aims to decrease the dose to the heart or lungs to reduce the risk of injury or long-term impact. This can be accomplished with both proton and photon treatments.

Quick Soap Box Moment: Television commercials by for-profit cancer centers, the internet, and sometimes the media will make claims that "proton therapy is safer" or "proton therapy does not damage the heart or lungs like photon therapy." What those statements should actually say is, "Proton therapy is safer than photon therapy was thirty years ago." Or "Proton therapy does not damage the heart or lungs like photon therapy used to do many years ago."

"I want the best!" We all do, right? The good news is, ladies, you've got options. You choose the brand of phone you buy, the brand of shoes you wear, what kind of car you like. Photons or protons.

In the end, what really is proton therapy for breast cancer? The answer is, an option.

Glossary

Adjuvant: treatment that isn't surgery; "add-on" treatment (i.e., radiation or chemo)

Adriamycin: big guns chemo; can be hard on the heart

Axilla: armpit

BRCA1 and BRCA2: genes that we all have; however, some people are born with a gene that is not functioning like it should, and this gives them an increased risk of some cancers (notably breast and ovarian cancer)

Carcinoma: cancer (arising from an epithelial origin)

Carbo/Taxol: in the breast cancer world, these guys like to travel together

Chemotherapy: that awful but pretty awesome stuff that poisons that cancer (but sometimes gets a little lost along the ways and gets some healthy cells too . . . enter: side effects)

Cisplatin: chemo that has something against the nerves (and I am not talking about being brave)

Compazine (Prochlorperazine): anti-nausea

DNA (deoxyribonucleic acid): the recipe for us!

Ductal Carcinoma in Situ (DCIS): breast cancer that is not supposed to leave the breast (it doesn't even leave the milk duct it started in)

Estrogen Receptor: 70 percent of all breast cancers have these guys, and they benefit you by being a target for therapy if you have them.

Grade: This is not your stage; this describes how the breast cancer cells look under the microscope.

HER2 Receptor: 30 percent of breast

cancers have this sucker, and it's a growth receptor. Luckily, there are two really great drugs specifically aimed to seek and destroy these breast cancer cells!

Herceptin: fancy drug to target those little beasties that have HER2 receptors on them; can be a bit hard on the heart

Local Regional Recurrence (LRR): cancer that comes back in the breast or armpit lymph nodes

Lymphedema: swelling due to increased fluid

Metastasis: cancer that has spread beyond the breast

Neoadjuvant: therapy that happens before surgery

Neuropathy: damage to nerves that can cause alteration in sensation (numb, tingly, etc.)

Oncotype Dx Score®: a genetic test performed on the tumor tissue to determine if you will benefit from chemotherapy

Perjeta: HER2 Receptor targeting drug—KAPOW!

Phenergan (Promethazine): anti-nausea med

Progesterone Receptor: If you are positive for this, great! We have a bulls-eye on the cancer and medications (that aren't chemo) to treat it!

Prognosis: This is a random percentage that really means nothing to you, girl. It's all or nothing 100 percent or 0 percent for each individual lady. But on the whole, most breast cancer has a good prognosis. Yay!

Radiation: X-rays that decrease the chance of getting breast cancer again in that breast.

Receptor: These are the satellite dishes that a breast cancer cell puts on its roof. It also acts like a bulls-eye for therapy!

Reglan (Metoclopramide): anti-nausea med

Stage: A number that attempts, but in no way actually helps, to predict your future.

Taxol (T) AKA Paclitaxel: chemotherapy that is derived from nature and has something against hair follicles.

Zofran (Ondansetron): anti-nausea med

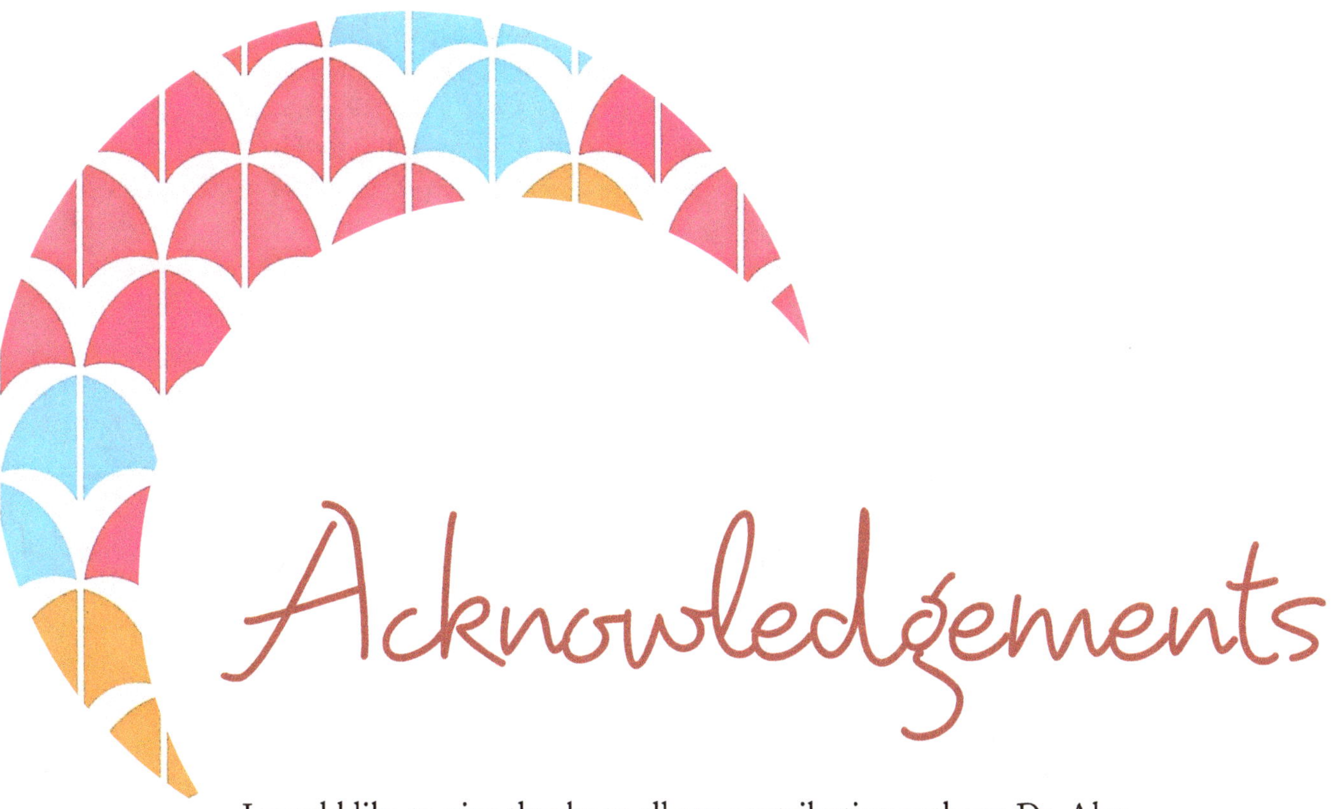

Acknowledgements

I would like to give thanks to all my contributing authors: Dr. Alan Hollingsworth, Dr. Maryann Martinovic, Dr. Lisa Spiguel, Dr. Astrid Morrison, Dr. David Schomas, Victoria Hand, and DeBorrah Carter. I would also like to acknowledge Janis Fultz and the patients that shared their personal thoughts. A special thank you to my initial audience that read through rough drafts and steered me in the right direction: my parents, Debora and Michael McCabe; Gillian Schoeneck; Marilyn Gilbaugh; and Abby Bova. Also, thanks to those who contributed images: Dr. Melanie Pearce, Astrid Morrison (again), and Dr. Michele Powers. Finally, to my copy editor, Jenna Love, who made this a polished written work.

About the Author

I was introduced to breast cancer at a very young age. My grandmother was diagnosed with inflammatory breast cancer at age fifty while living in Alaska. In order to receive neoadjuvant chemotherapy and enroll in clinical trials, she lived with my family in Southern California. My clearest memories of my grandma "mee-mee" were of her wearing headscarves and face masks. My father was in the Navy, and I grew up moving around the United States, gifted with the experience of meeting people from all walks of life. My mother was an elementary school teacher, and I spent hours tutoring and learning the value of thoughtful and clear communication. I went on to graduate college with degrees in Biochemistry and English with honors. My English honors thesis focused on the metaphors that breast cancer survivors used in their memoirs to understand and cope with their cancer diagnosis, their treatments, and the side effects. In preparation, I read every breast cancer memoir that I could find. I then completed medical school, general surgery residency, two years in a basic science research laboratory, and breast surgery fellowship with the goal of focusing on the treatment of women with breast cancer. My mother still talks about how wonderful my grandmother's doctors were. I grew up listening to just how important the relationship is between a woman and her doctor; and how, sometimes, that makes all the difference. I will always aim to be the little ray of sunshine in an otherwise stormy journey through breast cancer.

www.ingramcontent.com/pod-product-compliance
Lightning Source LLC
LaVergne TN
LVHW081259100826
845148LV00005B/921

9781737379331